# OCD IN CHILDREN
# AND ADOLESCENTS

# OCD
# in Children
# and Adolescents
## A Cognitive-Behavioral
## Treatment Manual

**John S. March, MD, MPH**
**Karen Mulle, BSN, MTS, MSW**

*Foreword by Edna B. Foa, PhD*

The Guilford Press
New York    London

© 1998 by John S. March and Karen Mulle
Published by The Guilford Press
A Division of Guilford Publications, Inc.
72 Spring Street, New York, NY 10012
http:\\www.guilford.com

Printed in the United States of America

This book is printed on acid-free paper.

Last digit is print number:    9  8  7  6  5

**Library of Congress Cataloging-in-Publication Data**

March, John S., MD.
    OCD in children and adolescents: a cognitive-behavioral
treatment manual / John S. March, Karen Mulle.
        p.    cm.
    Includes bibliographical references and index.
    ISBN 1-57230-242-9
    1. Obsessive-compulsive disorder in children—Treatment.
2. Obsessive-compulsive disorder in adolescence—Treatment.
3. Cognitive therapy for children.    4. Cognitive therapy for
teenagers.    I. Mulle, Karen.    II. Title.
RJ506.O25M37   1998
618.92'852270651—dc21                                    98-2637
                                                          CIP

*To our young patients*
*on whose courage this text rests*

Courage is not simply one of the virtues but
the form of every virtue at the testing point.
—C. S. Lewis

# Foreword

It was with great pleasure that I accepted the invitation to write a foreword for this excellent treatment manual for therapists in the delivery of cognitive-behavioral therapy (CBT) to children and adolescents with obsessive–compulsive disorder (OCD). It has long been recognized that CBT is the most effective psychotherapeutic approach to OCD in adults. Research dating back into the 1970s has demonstrated that the combination of exposure and response prevention has been highly effective in ameliorating OCD in adults suffering from the disorder (e.g., Kozak & Foa, 1997; Rachman & Hodgson, 1980). In comparison with CBT, the effect of medication is more moderate and fewer patients benefit from it. Moreover, the vast majority of patients who receive CBT continue to maintain their gains long after treatment has been completed, whereas many patients who are helped by medication relapse after their medication is discontinued. Recently, we have focused on how to adapt treatments developed and tested in research settings to the needs of clinicians and mental health providers (Kozak & Foa, 1997) and even to self-help programs (Foa & Wilson, 1991).

In the last few years it has become apparent that a large number of children and adolescents suffer from OCD and that children with OCD often become adults with OCD. Pharmaceutical companies have purposefully pursued pharmacological remedies for OCD, but until now there have been few published treatment resources specifically addressing how to implement effective cognitive-behavioral strategies with young patients. Thus, the need for a treatment program like the one in this book is very great. Dr. March and his colleagues have unparalleled experience using CBT to treat young persons with OCD, and this book represents the distillation of years of clinical wisdom and empirical study. This makes the book a superb addition to the growing literature on the cognitive-behavioral treatment of children, adolescents, and adults with anxiety disorders.

As this book attests, Dr. March's work on extending psychopharmacological and cognitive-behavioral treatments to children and adolescents with OCD is well known and sets the world standard in this area. Few clinical researchers take upon themselves the tedious but essential task of progressing systematically from pilot studies to controlled trials to wider dissemination to the clinical community. Hence, it was with great delight, first intellectual and then personal, that I began collaborating with Dr. March over 10 years ago. These collaborative endeavors have matured to the point that we are currently conducting an NIMH-funded comparative treatment outcome study at our two sites, Allegheny University of the Health Sciences in Philadelphia and Duke University in Durham, North Carolina. Using a volunteer sample of 120 (60 per site) 8- to 16-year-olds with a DSM-IV diagnosis of OCD, we are comparing the degree and durability of improvement obtained by treating patients with medication (a serotonin reuptake inhibitor), OCD-specific CBT, and a combination of medication and CBT. Having first compared the outcome of the treatment across the different treatment conditions, we then go on to assess treatment durability when treatment is withdrawn in responders. Once completed, our study should considerably advance the literature on the descriptive psychopathology and treatment of OCD in young persons.

Despite rapid progress, empirical evidence favoring CBT as a treatment for OCD in young persons remains relatively weak when compared to the ample evidence favoring CBT in adults. In the Center for the Study and Treatment of Anxiety in Philadelphia, we have used the program outlined in this book and compared it to an intensive program of CBT that we developed. The results showed that both programs are effective treatments for children and adolescents with OCD (Franklin et al., 1998). Yet much remains to be done. Future research needs to focus on the following: (1) controlled trials like the one that Dr. March and I are currently conducting comparing medication, CBT, and combination treatment to determine whether medication and CBT are synergistic or additive in their effects on OCD symptoms; (2) follow-up studies to evaluate relapse rates, including examining the utility of booster CBT in reducing relapse rates in patients treated with medication alone or in combination with CBT;

(3) component analyses, such as a comparison of exposure and response prevention to evaluate the relative contributions of specific treatment components to symptom reduction and treatment acceptability; (4) comparisons of individual- and family-based treatments to determine which is more effective in which children; (5) development of innovative treatment for OCD subtypes, such as obsessional slowness, primary obsessional OCD, and tic-like OCD, which do not respond as well to exposure and response prevention; (6) targeting treatment innovations to factors that constrain the application of CBT to patients with OCD, such as family dysfunction; and (7) exporting research treatments to divergent clinical settings and patient populations in order to judge the acceptability and effectiveness of CBT as a treatment for child, adolescent, and adult OCD in real-world settings.

Dr. March and his colleague Karen Mulle have performed a unique service in guiding this program of research from its inception over 10 years ago to the publication of what today is truly a master clinician's guide to the treatment of OCD in young persons. Ten years ago, such a publication seemed to many clinicians too large a task to be feasible. I am proud to have encouraged Dr. March to take up the challenge of making CBT developmentally appropriate to the needs of our youngest patients with OCD. These young persons and their families are the true beneficiaries of this remarkable text and the commitment to evidence-based psychiatric treatments on which it rests.

EDNA B. FOA, PHD
*Allegheny University*
*Philadelphia, PA*

## REFERENCES

Foa, E. B., & Wilson, R. (1991). *Stop obsessing! How to overcome your obsessions and compulsions*. New York: Bantam Doubleday Dell.

Franklin, M. E., Kozak, M. J., Cashman, L. A., Coles, M. E., Rheingold, A. A., & Foa, E. B. (1998). Cognitive-behavioral treatment of pediatric obsessive-compulsive disorder: An open clinical trial. *Journal of the American Academy of Child and Adolescent Psychiatry, 37*(4).

Kozak, M. J., & Foa, E. B. (1997). *Mastery of your obsessive compulsive disorder*. New York: Graywind.

Rachman, S., & Hodgson, R. (1980). *Obsessions and compulsions*. Englewood Cliffs, NJ: Prentice Hall.

# Preface

Some people never learn anything because they understand
everything too soon.

—*Alexander Pope*

One in 200 young persons suffers from obsessive–compulsive disorder
(OCD) at any given time. This means that there are three to four
youngsters with OCD in the average-size elementary school and up to
20 or 30 in a large urban high school. The purpose of this treatment
manual is to help reduce the suffering of these young persons and their
families.

## THE DEVELOPMENT OF THIS MANUAL

Cognitive-behavioral therapy (CBT), and especially exposure plus
response prevention (E/RP), has for some time been widely considered
an effective treatment for OCD in youth (Johnston & March, 1993;
Wolff & Rapoport, 1988). Ten years ago, practicing clinicians routinely complained that children refused to comply with behavioral
treatments, while parents justifiably complained that most clinicians
didn't know how to use CBT to treat OCD in young persons. In part,
these lamentations reflected the fact that research on children greatly
lagged behind that in adults (March, Johnson, & Greist, 1990). To
address this problem, in 1989, we began systematically to explore the
most effective way to deliver CBT to young persons with OCD. This
effort, which was a component in a more broadly conceived OCD

research program, led to the development of our treatment program, named "How I Ran OCD Off My Land©" by a young man who was one of our first treatment successes. This program was greatly revised and expanded into the current treatment manual.

In developing a treatment manual for pediatric OCD, our goals were simple:

- To encourage patient and parental compliance.
- To create a program suitable for a wide variety of clinical settings.
- To facilitate the empirical evaluation of OCD treatment, which will, we hope, lead to improvements in technique.

Many treatment manuals are suitable only for expert therapists working in research settings. However, we want to help real children in community treatment settings. We have therefore tried to incorporate many "clinical pearls" that, in our experience, make CBT practical and effective for young persons with OCD.

## WHO SHOULD USE THIS BOOK?

This book is designed to help clinicians treat children and adolescents with OCD, and also to some extent OC-spectrum disorders, such as trichotillomania. We have used this treatment protocol in children as young as 4 years old and in adults over age 50, so the basic principles are applicable across a broad range of ages and aptitudes. Therapists, like patients, have a variety of beliefs about the nature of the psychotherapeutic process. CBT falls under the purview of social learning theory. Since many mental health providers are not well versed in CBT or social learning theory, we provide sufficient theoretical background to help practitioners from other psychotherapy traditions, such as dynamic or family psychotherapy, make this transition.

## CLINICAL OUTCOMES

We assume from the outset that most patients will show moderate to marked improvement with treatment. While it would be wonderful if treatment always led to complete symptom remission, OCD is more often a chronic waxing and waning disorder, so that many youngsters need to return periodically for CBT booster sessions. Over time, the majority of children under our care improve to the point of being subclinically ill, which we define to mean that no one but the child knows that OCD is still around. Some reach this point with CBT alone; others require CBT and medications. Some get there in a few weeks; others take a year or more. About 30% remain clinically symptomatic despite our best efforts, but the great majority of these young persons still experience significant benefit from treatment. Very few fail to benefit at all or drop out of treatment. Since others have had similar results using "How I Ran OCD Off My Land" in their clinical settings, we feel confident that the treatment protocol outlined in this manual is ready for wider dissemination.

## ORGANIZATION OF THE BOOK

In writing this book, we tried to follow the same procedures that we use in our pediatric OCD treatment program at Duke University Medical Center. Like the treatment protocol itself, each chapter has a specific set of goals that build on the preceding chapters. The manual is organized as follows:

### Part I: Introduction

In Chapter 1, we review the varied symptomatic presentations and patterns of comorbidity found in pediatric OCD to set the stage for the implementation of treatment.

In Chapter 2, we describe the initial assessment protocol for pediatric OCD that we use in the Program in Child and Adolescent Anxiety Disorders at Duke University. Because vagueness is anathema to skillful CBT, it is essential that the child have a comprehensive, multimodal, multitrait evaluation before beginning treatment.

Chapter 3 provides an overview of the treatment protocol we will be describing in detail in Chapters 4–16. It also addresses logistical issues such as how to pace each session and when to check in with the patient by telephone.

### Part II: Treatment

Chapters 4 through 16 provide a session-by-session guide to the cognitive-behavioral treatment of pediatric OCD. The description of each session includes a statement of goals, procedures to meet those goals, and a means of evaluating the outcome. We also include tips for therapists and parents and discuss developmental considerations. In describing the interventions, we move frequently between the third person ("the therapist should . . .") and the first person ("we often use . . .") so that we present instructions both directly and by example.

## Part III: Troubleshooting

In Chapter 17, we discuss what to do when not everything goes smoothly. We review reasons why some youngsters seem only partially responsive or even nonresponsive to CBT and suggest solutions to these common therapeutic roadblocks.

Chapter 18 focuses on "special wrinkles" for managing subtypes of OCD that do not necessarily respond well to standard E/RP and may require supplemental treatment interventions.

In Chapters 19 and 20, we describe techniques for working with families and schools. These interventions are extremely important, since both families and teachers are often entangled in a child's OCD symptoms.

## Appendices

In Appendices I and II, we provide patient handouts and assessment forms that you may copy and use with your patients.

Appendix III provides a list of resources that can be very useful to both patients and clinicians, as well as educational material that you can copy and distribute to your patients and their families.

## Using This Manual

In writing this manual, we have generally used the word "child" to indicate a child or adolescent. However, where special age-related issues arise, we specify younger children or adolescents. It has been our goal to use clear, nontechnical language throughout the manual so that it would be accessible to therapists from a variety of back-grounds. We encourage those using this program to broaden their knowledge of the disorder by reading many other books on OCD treatment. We have provided tips and "clinical pearls" in every chapter. Although these are generally included in the description of the phase of treatment where they seem most likely to be useful, such tips might be helpful at any point in treatment. It is therefore important that therapists carefully read the book as a whole before starting treatment.

In developing this manual, we have seen and treated hundreds of children and adolescents and have provided more than 2,000 hours of hands-on therapy for OCD. Along the way, we have made plenty of mistakes and taken lots of therapeutic detours, most of which you can avoid by following this manual. Children and families react differently to OCD, and OCD varies tremendously in its manifestations, so feel free to improvise when circumstances dictate. Applying the methods described in this manual in a rigid and inflexible way can be just as destructive as failing to follow it at all. While we have included a large number of "clinical pearls," there is no substitute for experience. As mentioned above, the wise therapist will also want to review other books to supplement the current one.

Always remember that OCD is the adversary. The therapist who fails to keep the focus on OCD, for example, by attending unnecessarily to peer or family problems instead of the session goals, becomes an ally of OCD through complicity with antiexposure instructions. We have found that this is a common problem for inexperienced therapists or therapists coming from other psychotherapy traditions, especially play or family therapy. If you stay within a skills-based cognitive-behavioral framework, you will more often than not keep your patient cheerfully engaged in treatment until one day your services fortunately are no longer needed.

## ACKNOWLEDGMENTS

While it has been our good fortune to participate in the development and dissemination of CBT for pediatric OCD, many others also deserve credit. Most of all, we owe a special debt of gratitude to the many patients and their families who have taught us so much about pediatric OCD. With so much of mental health care still driven by ineffective relationship-oriented psychotherapies, it often seems to us that our patients and their parents are ahead of the field in their understanding of OCD as a neuropsychiatric disorder. Their thoughtful observations, cheerfulness in the face of OCD, and willingness to wonder along with us as we worked the kinks out of the treatment protocol have been both professionally helpful and personally rewarding. Above all, what drives our commitment to the work of treatment development is the pleasure of watching a child's enthusiasm for successfully "bossing" OCD increase as treatment proceeds. We thank our patients and their families for the privilege of helping them.

In the 1970s, when behavioral psychotherapy for OCD was still novel, Isaac Marks and his colleagues at the Institute for Psychiatry in London clearly demonstrated that exposure-based interventions worked for adults with OCD (Marks, Hodgson, & Rachman, 1975). Subsequently, gifted psychologists and psychiatrists—among them Lee Baer, Edna Foa, and John Greist—extended the reach of behavioral psychotherapy and systematized its application in adults. Our work is merely an extension of theirs. The National Institute of Mental Health group—Judy Rapoport, Henrietta Leonard, and Susan Swedo—readily shared their insights about pediatric OCD and encourage the development of CBT for young persons with this disorder. Jeff Schwartz, who along with Lew Baxter demonstrated that CBT for OCD changes the brain in a durable fashion, and members of the OCD Beliefs Workgroup inspired our approach to the cognitive components of treatment. Above all, Edna Foa and Michael Kozak have been inspiring and expert guides in helping us to extend the benefits of CBT to children and adolescents. Taken collectively, the work of these extraordinary clinician researchers powerfully influenced our thinking; their friendship and generosity have been equally important.

When we found it impossible to distribute our original treatment manual, "How I Ran OCD Off My Land," any longer, the Obsessive–Compulsive (OC) Foundation in Milford, Connecticut, took over distribution of the original manual which benefited many families and therapists. Amazingly, version 1.4 of the treatment manual has now been distributed to over 4,000 clinicians and patients in a dozen countries, and has been translated into several different languages. We expect that this current substantially revised and updated effort (version 3.0) will achieve much wider distribution. As the book took shape, the able and patient support of Kitty Moore, Senior Editor at The Guilford Press, has been invaluable. Her wise counsel and honest desire to see a wider dissemination of scientific knowledge are primary causes for the publication of this text. Reflecting their genuine commitment to bringing both CBT and medications to patients suffering from OCD, Solvay Pharmaceuticals, Inc., generously provided a small independent educational grant to help see the book through to completion.

To these friends and colleagues, and to others in the OCD community whose purpose has been to ease the suffering of children with OCD by pushing on the edge of scientific knowledge about the diagnosis and treatment of OCD, we are deeply grateful. Without you this book would not have been written.

There is, of course, much more to life than academia, and I (JSM) want to thank my wife, Kathleen, and my children, Matthew and Maggie, for their good humor as I put this volume together. Their love and support make all other things, including the varied tasks of academic life, possible. I (KM) want to thank my parents, who gave special encouragement and were model "cheerleaders" as I worked on this volume. I also thank my community of faith and extended family and friends who provide the ongoing love and support needed to see beauty and possibilities even in difficult situations.

Finally, as in most areas of psychiatry and psychology, controversy abounds. This book, while rich in information, will in some instances not do justice to the edge of the field, and the reader may not agree with everything we say. The errors of fact are ours; the controversies will eventually yield to good science. Our goal in producing this manual is to help children and adolescents with OCD lead more normal, happy, and productive lives. We hope we have achieved this goal.

JOHN S. MARCH
KAREN MULLE
*Durham, North Carolina*

# Contents

# Part One

# I INTRODUCTION

It wasn't raining when Noah built the arc.
—*Anonymous*

Part I sets the stage for treatment. In Chapter 1, we give an overview of pediatric obsessive–compulsive disorder (OCD) for those unfamiliar with it. In Chapter 2, we describe how to perform the accurate initial assessment that is critical to the implementation of cognitive–behavioral therapy (CBT). In Chapter 3, we provide an overview of the treatment protocol that will be described in detail in the second part of the manual. The reader who is already expert in the diagnosis and CBT of OCD may wish to peruse these first three chapters quickly, referring back to them only when more specific information is needed. Most readers, however, will profit from a careful reading of this material, as these chapters define the theoretical and practical framework within which CBT for pediatric OCD unfolds.

# Chapter 1

## Review
## of Pediatric OCD

The old mind–body distinction does nothing but get in our way. Both medications and psychotherapy are effective because they work on the brain.
— *Steve Hyman, MD, Director, National Institutes of Mental Health*

One in 200 young persons suffers from OCD (Flament, 1990); in many cases, the disorder severely disrupts academic, social, and vocational functioning (Leonard, Swedo, et al., 1993; Adams, Waas, March, & Smith, 1994). Among children and adolescents with OCD, few receive a correct diagnosis and even fewer receive appropriate treatment (Flament et al., 1988). This is unfortunate because effective cognitive-behavioral (March, Mulle, & Herbel, 1994) and pharmacological (Leonard, Lenane, & Swedo, 1993; March, Leonard, & Swedo, 1995) treatments are now available. Successful cognitive–beavioral therapy (CBT) for children and adolescents with OCD depends on understanding the illness as it presents in young persons. Therefore, in this chapter, we briefly describe the epidemiology, diagnostic criteria, phenomenology and natural history, neurobiology, and treatment of OCD. Interested readers may also wish to consult a more in-depth discussion of assessment issues (Goodman & Price, 1992; March & Albano, 1996); diagnosis and comorbidity (Swedo, Rapoport, Leonard, Lenane, & Cheslow, 1989; Cohen & Leckman, 1994); OCD in the school setting (Adams et al., 1994); spectrum disorders (Rapoport,

1991; Leonard, Lenane, Swedo, Rettew, & Rapoport, 1991; Swedo, 1993); natural history (Leonard, Swedo, et al., 1993); cognitive-behavioral psychotherapy (March, 1995; March, Mulle, & Herbel, 1994; March & Mulle, 1996); and pharmacotherapy (Leonard & Rapoport, 1989).

## DIAGNOSIS AND ASSESSMENT

### Epidemiology

As in the adult population, OCD is substantially more common in children and adolescents than was once thought, with a 6-month prevalence of approximately 1 in 200 children and adolescents—which means that 3 or 4 children in each elementary school and up to 20 teenagers in most average-sized high schools have OCD (Rutter, Tizard, & Whitmore, 1970). One-third to one-half of adults with OCD developed the disorder during childhood (Rasmussen & Eisen, 1990).

Among patients seen at the National Institute of Mental Health (NIMH), boys were more likely to have prepubertal onset, to have a family member with OCD or Tourette syndrome (TS), and to show tic-like symptoms. Girls were more likely to have onset during adolescence and to have more phobic symptoms (Swedo, Rapoport, Leonard, et al., 1989). While there are more boys among children with prepubertal onset, the ratio of males to females equalizes in adolescence (Flament et al., 1988).

For unclear reasons, OCD is more common in Caucasian than African American children in clinical samples, although epidemiological data suggest no differences in prevalence as a function of ethnicity or geographic region (Rasmussen & Eisen, 1992).

Unfortunately, children and adolescents with OCD often go unrecognized. In one epidemiological survey of high school students, only 4 of the 18 children found to have OCD were under professional care (Flament et al., 1988). Moreover, none of the 18, including the 4 children in mental health treatment, had been correctly identified as suffering from OCD, perhaps confirming Jenike's characterization of OCD as a "hidden epidemic" (Jenike, 1989). OCD may be underdiagnosed and undertreated because of factors related to the disorder itself (e.g., secretiveness and lack of insight), factors related to health care providers (e.g., incorrect diagnosis, lack of familiarity with or unwillingness to use proven treatments), and other factors (e.g., lack of access to treatment resources).

## DSM-IV Diagnostic Criteria

As described in the *Diagnostic and Statistical Manual of Mental Disorders* (DSM-IV), OCD is characterized by recurrent obsessions and/or compulsions that cause marked distress and/or interference in one's life (American Psychiatric Association, 1994). The DSM-IV diagnostic criteria for OCD include the following key features:

• An affected youngster must have either obsessions or compulsions, although the great majority have both. *Obsessions* are recurrent and persistent thoughts, images, or impulses that are ego-dystonic, intrusive and, for the most part, acknowledged as senseless. Obsessions are generally accompanied by distressing negative affects, such as fear, disgust, doubt, or a feeling of incompleteness.

• Like adults, young persons with OCD typically attempt to ignore, suppress, or neutralize obsessive thoughts and associated feelings by performing *compulsions*. Compulsions are repetitive, purposeful behaviors that are often performed according to certain rules or in a stereotyped fashion in order to temporarily neutralize or alleviate obsessions and the dysphoric affects that accompany them. Compulsions can be observable behaviors (e.g., washing) or covert mental acts (e.g., counting).

• Since OCD behaviors often occur in individuals without a disorder, DSM-IV specifies that the OCD symptoms must be distressing, time-consuming (taking more than an hour a day), or must significantly interfere with school, social activities, or important relationships.

• DSM-IV specifies that the obsessions are not simply excessive worries about real problems and that affected individuals must recognize that the obsessions originate within the mind. Also, *at some point in the illness*, the person must recognize that the obsessions or compulsions are excessive and unreasonable. Although most children and adolescents recognize the senselessness of OCD, this requirement that insight be preserved is waived for children. When someone of any age lacks insight into the senselessness of the obsessions and compulsions, the specifier "with poor insight" is included as part of the diagnosis.

• To differentiate OCD from other disorders, DSM-IV requires that the specific content of the obsessions not be related to another Axis I diagnosis (e.g., obsessions about food in someone with an eating disorder, guilty thoughts [ruminations] associated with depression).

## Symptoms

Common obsessions and compulsions seen in pediatric OCD patients are presented in Table 1.1. The most common obsessions in pediatric patients are fear of contamination, fear of harm to oneself and to other people, especially familiar people, and urges related to a need for symmetry or exactness. Corresponding compulsions in children are excessive washing and cleaning, followed by checking, counting, repeating, touching, and straightening (Swedo, Rapoport, Leonard, et al., 1989). Most children develop washing and checking rituals at some time during the course of the illness. OCD symptoms change over time, often with no clear pattern of progression, and many children have more than one OCD symptom at any one time. Consequently, many individuals will have experienced almost all the classic OCD symptoms by the end of adolescence (Rettew, Swedo, Leonard, Lenane, & Rapoport, 1992). Children who have only obsessions or only compulsions are extremely rare (Swedo, Rapoport, Leonard, et al., 1989), especially since the DSM-IV criteria now make a clear distinction between obsessions and mental rituals and compulsions, thereby reducing the number of patients with mental compulsions who would formerly have been misclassified as having only obsessions. A clinically useful and detailed symptom checklist accompanies the Yale–Brown Obsessive Compulsive Scale (YBOCS; Good-

**TABLE 1.1.** Typical OCD Symptoms

| Common obsessions | Common compulsions |
| --- | --- |
| • Contamination themes | • Washing |
| • Harm to self or others | • Repeating |
| • Aggressive themes | • Checking |
| • Sexual themes | • Touching |
| • Scrupulosity/religiosity | • Counting |
| • Forbidden thoughts | • Ordering/arranging |
| • Symmetry urges | • Hoarding |
| • Need to tell, ask, confess | • Praying |

man, Price, Rassmussen, Mazure, Fleischmann, et al., 1989) (see Appendix II).

## Developmental Factors

Most, if not all, children exhibit normal age-dependent obsessive–compulsive (OC) behaviors. For example, young children frequently like things done "just so" or insist on elaborate bedtime rituals (Gesell, Ames, & Ilg, 1974). Such behaviors can often be understood in terms of developmental issues involving mastery and control and are usually gone by middle childhood, to be replaced by collecting, hobbies, and focused interests. Clinically, more normal OC behaviors can often be discriminated from OCD on the basis of timing, content, and severity (Leonard, Goldberger, Rapoport, Cheslow, & Swedo, 1990). Developmentally sanctioned obsessive–compulsive behaviors occur early in childhood, are rare during adolescence, are common to large numbers of children, and are associated with mastery of important developmental transitions. In contrast, OCD occurs somewhat later, appears bizarre to adults and to other children, if not to the affected child, and always produces dysfunction rather than mastery. Note, however, that when OCD intersects culturally dependent beliefs, such as the definition of appropriate cleanliness or religious obligations, these simple rules may not hold.

## Comorbidity

Children with a variety of other psychiatric disorders may exhibit obsessions or ritualistic behaviors, which can complicate the diagnosis of OCD in some patients. In addition, more than one disorder may be diagnosed in a single patient, since the diagnosis of OCD is not exclusionary. Tic disorders, anxiety disorders, disruptive behavior disorders, and learning disorders are common in clinical (Riddle et al., 1990; Swedo, Rapoport, Leonard, et al., 1989) and epidemiological samples of children with OCD (Flament et al., 1988). Comorbid OC spectrum disorders (e.g., trichotillomania, body dysmorphic disorder) and habit disorders (e.g., nail biting) are also not clinically uncommon. A surprisingly small number of children exhibit signs of obsessive–compulsive personality disorder (OCPD), implying that OC personality traits, while overrepresented among children with OCD, are neither necessary nor sufficient for the diagnosis (Swedo, Rapoport, Leonard, et al., 1989).

## Neuropsychology

As with adults, children and adolescents with OCD frequently exhibit subtle neurological (Denckla, 1989) and neuropsychological (Cox, Fedio, & Rapoport, 1989) problems, which often involve relative weakness in nonverbal as contrasted to verbal reasoning skills. In turn, deficits in nonverbal reasoning skills place children at risk for specific learning problems, such as dysgraphia, dyscalculia, poor expressive written language, and reduced processing speed and efficiency. While some have speculated that these neurocognitive impairments may adversely affect the outcome of pharmacotherapy for OCD (Hollander et al., 1990; March, Johnston, Jefferson, et al., 1990), others have found no such association (Swedo, Leonard, & Rapoport, 1990; Leonard & Rapoport, 1989). More importantly, children with learning style differences present a special problem in differential therapeutics. For example, a child slowed down by tracing rituals must be distinguished from the youngster slowed down by dysgraphia and poor expressive written language skills.

## OCD Is a Neuropsychiatric Disorder

Successful treatment of OCD with serotonin reuptake inhibitors (SRIs) quickly led to a neurobehavioral explanation for OCD—the "serotonin hypothesis" (reviewed in Barr, Goodman, Price, McDougle, & Charney, 1992). Later, phenomenological similarities between obsessive–compulsive symptoms (washing, evening, picking, and licking) coupled with studies of trichotillomania led to the hypothesis that, in some patients, OCD is a "grooming behavior gone awry" (Swedo, 1989). The following evidence supports a neuropsychiatric model of OCD:

- Family genetic studies suggesting that OCD and TS may, in some cases, represent alternate expressions of the same gene(s), may represent different genes, or may arise spontaneously (Pauls, Towbin, Leckman, Zahner, & Cohen, 1986; Pauls, Alsobrook, Goodman, Rasmussen, & Leckman, 1995).
- Neuroimaging studies implicating abnormalities in circuits linking basal ganglia to cortex (Swedo, Schapiro, et al., 1989; Rauch et al., 1994), with these circuits "responding" to either cognitive-behavioral or pharmacological treatment with an SRI (Baxter et al., 1992).
- Neurotransmitter and neuroendocrine abnormalities in child-

hood-onset OCD (Swedo & Rapoport, 1990; Hamburger, Swedo, Whitaker, Davies, & Rapoport, 1989).

Particularly relevant among these lines of evidence is the relationship between OCD and TS (Cohen & Leckman, 1994). It is now well documented that there is an increased rate of tic disorders in individuals with OCD; the converse is also true (Pauls et al., 1995). Also, in systematic family genetic studies of probands with TS or other tic disorders, first-degree relatives show an increased rate of both tic disorders and OCD (Pauls et al., 1986), while there have been similar findings in first-degree relatives of OCD probands (Leonard et al., 1992). Pauls et al. (1995) have also found that early onset may indicate a greater degree of genetic vulnerability. For a more detailed discussion of these and related topics, refer to the following reviews: Swedo and Rapoport (1990), Rapoport, Swedo, and Leonard (1992), Cohen and Leckman (1994), and March, Leonard, and Swedo (in press).

## Pediatric Autoimmune Neuropsychiatric Disorder Associated with Strep (PANDAS)

In a subgroup of children, OCD symptoms may develop or be exacerbated in the context of a Group A beta hemolytic streptococcal infection (GABHS)—"strep throat." OC symptoms are not uncommon in pediatric patients with Sydenham's chorea, which represents a neurological variant of rheumatic fever (RF). Sydenham's patients display involuntary tic-like writhing movements that usually involve the extremities and, less often, the facial muscles. OCD is far more common in rheumatic fever patients when chorea is present (Swedo, Rapoport, Cheslow, et al., 1989). Sydenham's chorea is believed to represent an autoimmune inflammation of the basal ganglia triggered by antistreptococcal antibodies (Kiessling, Marcotte, & Culpepper, 1994). For this reason, Swedo and colleagues speculated that OCD in the context of Sydenham's chorea may provide a medical model for both OCD and tic disorders (Swedo et al., 1993). In this model, antineuronal antibodies formed against group A beta-hemolytic strep cell wall antigens cross react with basal ganglia neural tissue, resulting in the development of OCD or tic symptoms. This theory suggests that when there is an acute onset or dramatic exacerbation of OCD or tic symptoms, the clinician should promptly investigate for a Group A strep infection, especially since immunomodulatory treatments, including antibiotic therapies, may benefit selected patients (Allen, Leonard, & Swedo, 1995; Swedo, Leonard, & Kiessling, 1994).

## TREATMENT

Though OCD may be the primary diagnosis, young persons with OCD vary considerably with respect to the specific nature and severity of their OC symptoms, the range of comorbid psychopathology, and the impact of the disorder on the child and family. Every youngster with OCD thus warrants a comprehensive individualized diagnostic assessment, including OCD symptoms, comorbidity, and psychosocial factors. In addition to targeting OCD symptoms, treatment planning also must consider the presence of comorbidity, such as depression or disruptive disorders; the child's developmental level, temperament, and level of adaptive functioning; and the family context within which OCD occurs and the treatment will take place. In this context, both the patient and family should participate to the greatest extent possible in the development of an individualized treatment plan.

### Cognitive-Behavioral Psychotherapy

In reviewing the psychoanalytic understanding of OCD, Esman noted that insight-oriented psychotherapy has, at best, proven disappointing in ameliorating OCD symptoms (Esman, 1989). Although it has been argued that some OCD symptoms have underlying dynamic meaning, it is doubtful that specific OCD symptoms really represent derivatives of intrapsychic conflicts, since a finite number of OCD symptoms that occur in a typical pattern are universally experienced. Moreover, there is no reason to suggest that OCD patients are any more conflicted about sexual matters than other psychiatric patients (Staebler, Pollard, & Merkel, 1993).

In contrast, CBT is increasingly described as the psychotherapeutic treatment of choice for children, adolescents, and adults with OCD (Berg, Rapoport, & Wolff, 1989; Wolff & Wolff, 1991). Unlike other psychotherapies that have been applied to OCD, CBT for OCD is based on a logically consistent and compelling relationship between the disorder, the treatment, and the specified outcome (Foa & Kozak, 1985). CBT has long been demonstrated to be a remarkably effective and durable treatment for adults with OCD (Dar & Greist, 1992); likewise, CBT can help the child to internalize a strategy for resisting OCD, which depends on a clear understanding of the disorder within a medical framework. While periodic "booster" sessions may be required, those who are successfully treated with CBT alone tend to stay well (March, 1995). Moreover, while relapse commonly follows medication discontinuation in OCD, March et al. (1994) found that improvement persisted in six of nine responders following withdrawal of medication, providing limited support for the hypothesis that behavioral therapy inhibits relapse when medications are discontinued.

## Pharmacotherapy

The medications most commonly used to treat OCD are the serotonin reuptake inhibitors (SRIs). These include the tricyclic antidepressant (TCA) clomipramine, which is an SRI, and the selective serotonin reuptake inhibitors (SSRIs), fluoxetine, fluvoxamine, paroxetine, and sertraline. SRIs have been clearly shown to be effective in adults with OCD (Greist et al., 1990; Jenike, 1992); studies of pediatric OCD patients suggest that these medications will be similarly helpful for children (for reviews, see Rapoport, Swedo, & Leonard, 1992; March, Leonard, & Swedo, 1995.

Of the SRIs, clomipramine has received the most study in the pediatric population. In initial studies, clomipramine was reported to be significantly superior to placebo (Flament et al., 1985) and to desipramine (Leonard, Lenane, et al., 1991). The results of an 8-week multicenter, double-blind, parallel comparison of clomipramine versus placebo in 1989 led to FDA approval of clomipramine for the treatment of OCD in children and adolescents age 10 and older (De-Veaugh-Geiss et al., 1992). Notable findings from this study included: (1) little or no placebo effect; (2) clinical effects beginning, on average, at 3 weeks and leveling off at 10 weeks; and (3) a 37% reduction in OCD symptoms as measured on the YBOCS, which corresponded to markedly to moderately improved on a measure of global improvement; conversely, fewer than 20% of the study participants fell below the threshold for a clinical diagnosis of OCD, suggesting that, while medication is helpful, it is not a panacea for most children.

The side effects of clomipramine seen in children were comparable to (but typically milder than) those seen in adult trials (Katz, DeVeaugh, & Landau, 1990; Leonard et al., 1989) and are primarily related to the anticholinergic, antihistaminic, and alpha-blocking properties of clomipramine. Table 1.2 contrasts the side effects typically seen with clomipramine with those of the SSRIs. The most common side effects of clomipramine in adults are cardiovascular, anticholinergic, and sexual side effects, and weight gain; the side

**TABLE 1.2.** Medication Side Effects

| Side effect | Drug(s) *less* likely to cause | Drug(s) *more* likely to cause |
| --- | --- | --- |
| Cardiovascular | SSRIs | Clomipramine |
| Sedation | SSRIs | Clomipramine |
| Insomnia | Clomipramine | SSRIs |
| Anticholinergic | SSRIs | Clomipramine |
| Weight gain | SSRIs | Clomipramine |
| Sexual | SSRIs (but still common) | Clomipramine |
| Akathisia | Clomipramine | SSRIs |
| Nausea/diarrhea | Clomipramine | SSRIs |

*Note.* From March, Frances, et al. (1997). Copyright 1997 by Expert Knowledge Systems, LLC. Reprinted by permission.

effects seen in children and adolescents are similar to those seen in adults. While long-term maintenance treatment with clomipramine does not seem to produce any unexpected adverse reactions (De-Veaugh-Geiss et al., 1992; Leonard, Swedo, et al., 1991), tachycardia and slightly increased PR, QRS, and QT-corrected intervals on the electrocardiogram have been found. Given the potential for TCA-related cardiotoxic effects, pretreatment and periodic electrocardiographic and therapeutic drug monitoring is warranted (Schroeder, Mullin, Elliott, & Steiner, 1989; Elliott & Popper, 1991; Leonard, Meyer, et al., 1995).

Although all the SSRIs are likely to be effective treatments for OCD in children and adolescents (Rapoport, Leonard, Swedo, & Lenane, 1993; March, Leonard, et al., 1995), there have been fewer systematic trials of these medications in younger patients. Fluoxetine has shown benefit in a one controlled trial in children and adolescents (Riddle et al., 1992); sertraline and fluvoxamine have shown benefit in open studies in children and adolescents (Cook, Charak, Trapani, & Zelko, 1994; Apter, Ratzioni, & King, 1994). Large multicenter registration trials of fluvoxamine and sertraline in children and adolescents have been completed, and both drugs appear to be effective (Riddle et al., 1996; March, Biederman, Wolkow, Safferman, & Group, 1997). The most common side effects of the SSRIs are hyperarousal, nausea/diarrhea, and sexual side effects (see Table 1.2); the side effect profile of the SSRIs in children is identical to that seen in adults.

There is considerable variance in the response to medication, and the therapist should prepare both child and parents for this. Approximately one-third of patients may fail to respond to monotherapy with a given SRI (DeVeaugh-Geiss et al., 1992), and the likelihood of achieving a response drops considerably after a third SRI trial. Additionally, since a substantial minority of patients will not respond until after 8 or even 12 weeks of treatment (DeVeaugh-Geiss, Katz, Landau & Moroz, 1991; Goodman, Price, Rasmussen, Delgado, et al., 1989; March, Leonard, et al., 1995), it is important to wait at least 8, and preferably 10, weeks before changing medications, adopting high dose strategies, or adding a second medication to the child's treatment regimen (March, Frances, Carpenter, & Kahn, 1997).

When a child does not respond or responds only partially to the first medication, it is sometimes useful to augment the SRI with a second medication (Leonard & Rapoport, 1989; Jenike & Rauch, 1994). However, only clonazepam and haloperidol have shown benefit as augmenting agents (Pigott, L'Heureux, & Rubenstein, 1992; McDougle et al., 1994; Leonard, Topol, et al., 1995). Given the risk of physiological dependence with clonazepam and extrapyramidal side effects with conventional antipsychotics, clonazepam should probably be restricted to patients with high levels of anxiety and haloperidol to those with tics or thought disorder symptoms. Furthermore, since concomitant CBT may be the most powerful augmenting treatment in patients who are unresponsive to medication (March et al., 1994), complex medication strategies for OCD should be considered only for those patients who have not done well with high-quality CBT combined with an SRI.

## Combined Treatment

Most medical illnesses, including psychiatric illnesses, require pharmacological and/or psychosocial treatments that have been empirically demonstrated to be effective for the target symptoms of the disorder. Treatments should also help patients and their families cope with what cannot yet be cured (March, Mulle, Stallings, Erhardt, & Conners, 1995). The care of the diabetic patient provides a useful model: Treatment involves medication with insulin or oral hypoglycemics (depending on the subtype of the disorder); diet and exercise to control blood sugar using behavior modification; and interventions, such as diabetic foot care, to help with the sometimes unavoidable effects of the illness. Treatment for OCD involves CBT and medication with an SRI, alone or in combination, plus supportive individual, group, and family interventions.

Clinically, pharmacotherapy and CBT work well together, and clinicians generally believe that most children with OCD require or would be likely to obtain more benefit from a combined treatment approach (Piacentini et al., 1992; Johnston & March, 1993). However, as yet no controlled studies have been published comparing CBT, medication, and their combination in children and adolescents with OCD. In one study of protocol-driven CBT with patients who responded only partially to medication, the average magnitude of improvement on the YBOCS was noticeably greater (50%) than that usually seen with medications alone (30–40%) (March et al., 1994). While these findings suggest that combination treatment may have an advantage over pharmacotherapy alone, additional research is clearly needed to discover the relative merits of CBT and SRIs used alone or in combination for specific subgroups of patients.

## Treatment Planning Using the Expert Consensus Guidelines for the Treatment of OCD

Although an insufficient number of mental health providers are trained in CBT today, this will almost certainly change as psychiatry increasingly embraces the disease management model, which relies upon practice guidelines similar to those used throughout the rest of medicine. Practice guidelines help clinicians choose effective treatments that are compatible with the managed care objective of cost-effective quality care—using them is, in a sense, like having an expert at your elbow to provide answers to questions such as these:

- When do you use behavior therapy in children and adolescents with OCD?
- When do you use drug therapy?
- Is there an advantage to combining CBT and drug therapy?
- When should you change course in treatment?
- Once your patient is better, what should you do?

The *Expert Consensus Treatment Guidelines for Obsessive–Compulsive Disorder* (March, Frances, et al., 1997), which are based on a survey of 69 experts on OCD, provide answers to these and other

**TABLE 1.3.** Executive Summary A from Expert Consensus Treatment Guidelines for OCD

---

A. Consensus recommendations for first line treatments by clinical situation

---

*Selecting the initial treatment strategy and the sequence of treatments*
  Age specific considerations
  - Prepubescent children: CBT first for milder or more severe OCD
  - Adolescents: CBT first for milder OCD; CBT + SRI for more severe OCD
  - Adults: CBT first for milder OCD; CBT + SRI or SRI alone first for more severe OCD

  Considerations based on overall efficacy, speed, and durability of treatment
  - Milder OCD: CBT alone; or CBT + SRI
  - More severe OCD: CBT + SRI

  Considerations based on tolerability and patient acceptability
  - Milder OCD: CBT alone; or CBT + SRI
  - More severe OCD: CBT + SRI; or SRI alone

*Selecting CBT strategy*
  Obsessions and compulsions ──────┬──▶ E/RP
                                   └──▶ E/RP + CT

  *Tailoring treatment for specific symptoms*
  Contamination fears, symmetry ──────▶ E/RP
    rituals, counting/repeating,
    hoarding, aggressive urges
  Scrupulosity and moral guilt, ──────▶ CT
    pathological doubt

*Intensity of CBT*
  - Gradual (i.e., weekly): recommended for most patients (usually 13–20 sessions)
  - Intensive (i.e., daily): recommended when speed is of the essence or for patients who have not responded to gradual CBT or who have extremely severe symptoms

*Selecting a specific medication: use a serotonin reuptake inhibitor (SRI)*
  - Fluvoxamine
  - Fluoxetine
  - Clomipramine
  - Sertraline
  - Paroxetine

  *Recommendations for timing*
  - Inadequate response to average SRI dose: push to maximum dose in 4–9 weeks from start of treatment
  - Inadequate response after 4–6 additional weeks at maximum dose: switch to another SRI

*Treatment resistance*
  If no response or partial response ──────▶ Add an SRI; add more CBT
    to CBT alone                                with changes in approach

*(cont.)*

**TABLE 1.3** (*cont.*)

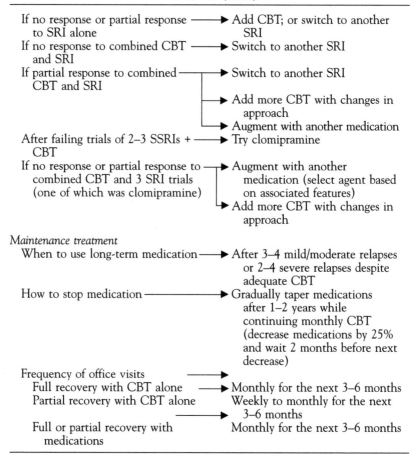

If no response or partial response ⟶ Add CBT; or switch to another
to SRI alone                                                SRI

If no response to combined CBT ⟶ Switch to another SRI
and SRI

If partial response to combined ⟶ Switch to another SRI
CBT and SRI

         ⟶ Add more CBT with changes in
            approach

         ⟶ Augment with another medication

After failing trials of 2–3 SSRIs + ⟶ Try clomipramine
CBT

If no response or partial response to ⟶ Augment with another
combined CBT and 3 SRI trials                    medication (select agent based
(one of which was clomipramine)               on associated features)
         ⟶ Add more CBT with changes in
            approach

*Maintenance treatment*

When to use long-term medication ⟶ After 3–4 mild/moderate relapses
          or 2–4 severe relapses despite
          adequate CBT

How to stop medication ⟶ Gradually taper medications
          after 1–2 years while
          continuing monthly CBT
          (decrease medications by 25%
          and wait 2 months before next
          decrease)

Frequency of office visits ⟶
  Full recovery with CBT alone ⟶ Monthly for the next 3–6 months
  Partial recovery with CBT alone    Weekly to monthly for the next
          ⟶ 3–6 months
  Full or partial recovery with          Monthly for the next 3–6 months
  medications

*Note.* CBT = cognitive-behavioral therapy; CT = cognitive therapy; E/RP = exposure/response prevention; SRI (serotonin reuptake inhibitor) refers to the five compounds clomipramine, fluoxetine, fluvoxamine, paroxetine, and sertraline; SSRI (selective SRI) refers to all but clomipramine. From March, Frances, et al. (1997). Copyright 1997 by Expert Knowledge Systems, LLC. Reprinted by permission.

questions about the treatment of OCD across the life span. A summary of the recommendations from the guidelines are shown in Tables 1.3 and 1.4 and Figures 1.1 and 1.2. The experts recommended CBT or CBT plus medication as the preferred treatment for pediatric OCD, with CBT alone preferred in younger patients and those with milder symptoms. These guidelines also include recommendations for managing the patient who responds poorly to initial treatment, choosing

**TABLE 1.4.** Executive Summaries B–D from Expert Consensus Treatment
Guidelines for OCD

B. Consensus recommendations for first-line psychosocial treatments

*Cognitive-behavioral therapy*
  For OCD, CBT involves E/RP combined with CT
  • When available, CBT is likely to be used for every patient with OCD
    except those who have very severe symptoms or who are unwilling to
    participate in CBT
  • Add when patient has been a nonresponder or partial responder to SRI
    alone
  • Use alone if patient is intolerant to side effects of medication. is
    pregnant. or has a medical condition that contraindicates medication
  • Use when there is comorbidity with other psychiatric disorders for
    which CBT may be helpful, especially if modified for the comorbid
    disorder

*Exposure plus response prevention*
  Especially helpful for contamination or other fears, symmetry rituals,
  counting/repeating, hoarding, aggressive urges

*Cognitive therapy*
  Especially helpful for scrupulosity, moral guilt, and pathological doubt

*Treatment format and intensity*
  • Format: Individual weekly therapy sessions combined with homework or
    therapist-assisted out-of-office (in vivo) techniques. Consider adding
    family therapy when appropriate.
  • Frequency: 13–20 sessions typically required to treat an uncomplicated
    OCD patient.
  • Intensity: Gradual, i.e., weekly: recommended for most patients.
    Intensive, i.e., daily: recommended when speed is of the essence or
    patients have not responded to gradual CBT or have very severe
    symptoms.
  • Maintenance schedule: Monthly booster sessions for 3–6 months

C. Consensus recommendations for first-line somatic treatments

*Selective serotonin reuptake inhibitors (fluvoxamine, fluoxetine, sertraline, paroxetine)*
  • Combine with CBT or use alone in adults with moderate to severe
    symptoms
  • Add when no response or partial response to CBT alone
  • Use before clomipramine and whenever anticholinergic, cardiovascular,
    sexual, sedative, or weight gain side effects are a concern
  • Use when there is comorbidity with other psychiatric disorders for
    which an SSRI may be helpful

*Clomipramine*
  • After 2–3 failed SSRI trials
  • Augment SSRI in partially responsive or nonresponsive patient
  • Less likely than SSRIs to cause insomnia, akathisia, nausea, or diarrhea
  • Use when there is comorbidity with other psychiatric disorders for
    which a TCA may be helpful                                      *(cont.)*

**TABLE 1.4** (*cont.*)

D. Consensus recommendations for OCD complicated by comorbid illness

| *Comorbidity* | |
| --- | --- |
| Pregnancy | CBT alone |
| Heart disease | CBT alone; or CBT + SSRI |
| Renal disease | CBT alone; or CBT + SSRI |
| Tourette syndrome | CBT + conventional antipsychotic + SRI |
| Attention-deficit/hyperactivity disorder | CBT + SSRI + psychostimulant |
| Panic disorder or social phobia | CBT + SSRI |
| Major depressive disorder | CBT + SRI (start SRI first for severe symptoms) |
| Bipolar disorder (I or II) | CBT + mood stabilizer alone; or CBT + mood stabilizer + SRI |
| Opposition/conduct/antisocial disorder | CBT + family therapy +SRI |
| Schizophrenia | SRI + neuroleptic |

*Note.* CBT = cognitive-behavioral therapy; CT = cognitive therapy; E/RP = exposure/response prevention; SRI (serotonin reuptake inhibitor) refers to the five compounds clomipramine, fluoxetine, fluvoxamine, paroxetine, and sertraline; SSRI (selective SRI) refers to all but clomipramine; TCA = tricyclic antidepressant. From March, Frances, et al. (1997). Copyright 1997 by Expert Knowledge Systems, LLC. Reprinted by permission.

therapies for treatment refractory patients, selecting among medications and CBT techniques, maintenance therapy, discontinuation of medications, and managing medical and psychiatric comorbidity.

The "Guide for Patients and Families" that was developed as part of the *Expert Consensus Guidelines* summarizes the experts' recommendations and is included in Appendix III.

## Predicting the Outcome of Treatment

Comorbid schizotypy (Baer et al., 1992) and tic disorders (McDougle et al., 1994) can interfere with the treatment of OCD and may indicate the need to add an antipsychotic to the treatment regimen. However, no specific predictors of treatment outcome in pediatric OCD have been identified. Patient age, sex, and socioeconomic status did not predict response to treatment in the NIMH (Leonard et al., 1989) and CIBA studies (DeVeaugh-Geiss et al., 1992) or predict relapse when desipramine was substituted for clomipramine (Leonard, Swedo, et al., 1991). Nor did characteristics of the specific OCD

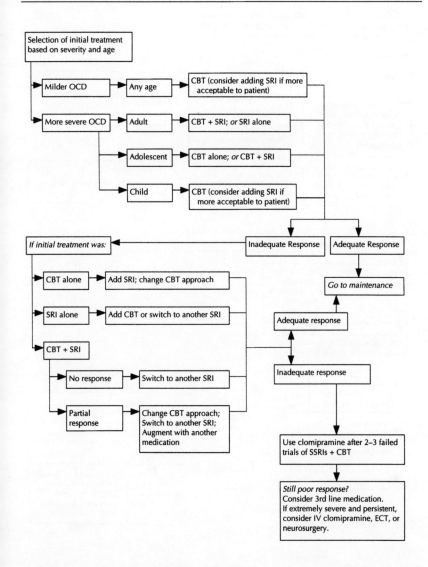

**FIGURE 1.1.** Treatment algorithm from Expert Consensus Treatment Guidelines for OCD: Overall strategies for acute phase treatment of OCD. From March, Frances, et al. (1997) Copyright 1997 by Expert Knowledge Systems, LLC. Reprinted by permission.

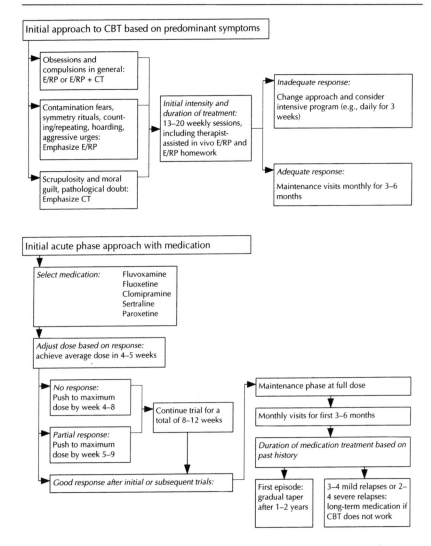

**FIGURE 1.2.** Treatment algorithm from Expert Consensus Treatment Guidelines for OCD: Tactics for duration and intensity of treatment during acute and maintenance phases. From March, Frances, et al. (1997) Copyright 1997 by Expert Knowledge Systems, LLC. Reprinted by permission.

presentation, such as initial severity, duration of symptoms, and symptom pattern, predict response to treatment (Leonard et al., 1989). Children who can acknowledge that their obsessions are senseless and that their rituals are distressing may be better candidates for CBT than those who don't, although lack of insight does not necessarily render CBT ineffective (Kettl & Marks, 1986).

Clinically, the presence of other comorbid disorders, especially oppositional defiant disorder or conduct disorder, appears to predict treatment resistance to both pharmacotherapy and CBT, but this hypothesis has not yet been tested in a controlled study with children with OCD. Similarly, while family dysfunction is neither necessary nor sufficient for the onset of OCD (Lenane, 1989), families affect and are affected by OCD; a family that is excessively critical and overinvolved may exacerbate OCD whereas a calm supportive family may improve the outcome of treatment (Hibbs et al., 1991). Table 1.4 summarizes expert consensus recommendations for combining treatments in the presence of comorbid conditions. See also Chapter 18, "Special Wrinkles," for a more detailed discussion of this issue.

## SUMMARY

OCD is a neurobehavioral disorder characterized by dysregulation in the circuits that link the frontal cortex of the brain to the basal ganglia. The disorder is substantially influenced by serotonergic and perhaps dopaminergic neurotransmission. Although current treatments cannot generally *cure* OCD, given a correct diagnosis and the skillful combination of a serotonin reuptake inhibitor and OCD-specific cognitive-behavioral psychotherapy, most children can be helped to resume a more normal developmental trajectory and thus to live a happier, more productive life.

# Chapter 2

## Assessing OCD

*I get a lot of answers, but no one ever asks the right questions.*

*—Dennis the Menace*

The nature and impact of OCD in children and adolescents varies widely. Comorbid psychiatric illnesses, such as social phobia, attention-deficit/hyperactivity disorder (ADHD), and tic disorders, are often present and pose complex problems for the therapist. Thus, an accurate and compassionate assessment of the pediatric patient with OCD, including a careful search for comorbid conditions that could complicate treatment, is essential to the skillful treatment of these patients (Wolff & Wolff, 1991; Thyer, 1991; March & Albano, 1996). It is also important to monitor the process and outcome of treatment using measures that sample specific symptom domains (e.g., washing), functional domains (e.g., home or school), and symptomatic distress during exposure (e.g., subjective units of discomfort—SUDS) (March, 1995). Since many patients improve considerably but far fewer become symptom free, global measures of impairment (e.g., Clinical Global Impairment Scale; NIMH Global Obsessive–Compulsive [OC] Scale; see Appendix II) and improvement (e.g., Clinical Global Improvement Scale) may help elucidate the need for ongoing or additional treatment. Methods of assessing treatment outcome are described in Chapter 3 ("Overview of Treatment") and in the chapters describing

---

This chapter is adapted from March, Mulle, Stallings, Erhardt, and Conners (1995). Copyright 1995 by The Guilford Press. Adapted by permission.

individual treatment sessions in Part II of this manual. In this chapter, we describe the initial evaluation we use in the Program for Child and Adolescent Anxiety Disorders at Duke University Medical Center.

## THE ASSESSMENT PROCESS

### Goals of the Initial Evaluation

Most mental health clinicians are familiar with treatments that emphasize issues related to the patient's history and current relationships. In contrast to these "story oriented" approaches, the cognitive-behavioral treatment of pediatric OCD involves adopting a disease management model in which the clinician acts as a coach to teach the patient a set of adaptive coping strategies for reducing OCD symptoms. Establishing targets for successful coping is a task in differential therapeutics—defining different treatments that are appropriate for differing treatment targets. This task can be seen as something like a game of pick-up sticks. The clinician has to correctly identify the targets of treatment (the sticks), pair them with target-specific treatments—in this case, exposure-based interventions—and sequence these interventions appropriately (pick up the sticks in the proper order) to help the patient get better.

How does the process of making a diagnosis of OCD fit this picture? Initially, the clinician is aware only of the presenting complaint, say declining school performance. Given the relatively rarity of OCD compared to depression or one of the disruptive behaviors disorders, just on the basis of probability it is likely that OCD is not the primary disorder—though it still might be! Nevertheless, because children are often secretive about their OCD symptoms, specific questions about OCD, including examples, should be a part of every diagnostic assessment.

Let's assume for the sake of discussion, however, that an OCD symptom, say excessive handwashing, is the reason that the child is coming for an evaluation. The clinician's first task then is to confirm OCD as the primary diagnosis and to rule out other diagnoses, such as depression or panic disorder, that share features with OCD. The process is directly analogous to that used by a cardiologist seeing a patient with chest pain in the emergency room. The primary hypothesis here is myocardial infarction or unstable angina, an impending heart attack. To rule out other sources of cardiac pain, such as chest wall pain, gallbladder disease, and other medical conditions, and not incidentally, panic disorder, the cardiologist systematically reviews the symptoms of these disorders. Having established the diagnosis of an acute myocardial infarction, the cardiologist then devises a treatment plan tailored to the specific needs of his patient.

Likewise, the mental health provider, after establishing a primary diagnosis of OCD and documenting complicating comorbid conditions, moves on to develop a specific treatment plan that targets those OCD symptoms that are unique to the patient (see Figure 2.1). The process begins with establishing a likely but still hypothetical diagnosis. The clinician then systematically assesses each DSM-IV diagnostic category. Finally, the clinician reaches a molecular understanding of the patient's OCD symptoms and of how well the patient has coped with them. The process of establishing a set of DSM diagnoses involves systematically grouping together clusters of symptoms that may later be targets of treatment, whether for OCD or for complicating comorbid conditions. In the rest of the chapter, we will examine in detail the process of moving from the presenting complaint to a DSM-IV diagnosis or diagnoses. In subsequent chapters, we will discuss how to tailor treatment to the patient's specific OCD symptoms.

### Referral

Table 2.1 lists the primary diagnoses that commonly result in referral to the Program in Child and Adolescent Anxiety Disorders (PCAAD)

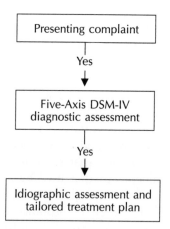

**FIGURE 2.1.** Assessment and treatment process.

**TABLE 2.1.** Primary Diagnoses
Referred to Our Anxiety
Disorders Program

Obsessive–Compulsive Disorder
Separation Anxiety Disorder
Generalized Anxiety Disorder
Generalized Social Phobia
Specific Social Phobia
Selective Mutism
Panic Disorder
Specific Phobias
Trichotillomania (hair pulling)
Posttraumatic Stress Disorder
"School Phobia"

at Duke University Medical Center. These disorders are similar to those seen in other pediatric anxiety disorders programs. Because we are a subspecialty clinic, many patients and their families come to us directly seeking treatment specifically for OCD. In fact, a good way to expand your practice is to become a referral site for patients who require specialized expertise. Other referral sources include physicians, psychologists, other mental health professionals, schools, the Obsessive–Compulsive Foundation (OCF), and local patient support groups. By the time they reach us, many of our patients are remarkably sophisticated regarding the diagnosis and treatment of anxiety disorders in youth. For example, we have recently seen several patients with OCD who learned about our program on one of several OCD web sites on the Internet.

## Telephone Contact

In some programs, a secretary or research assistant determines whether the referral is appropriate, discusses financial considerations, and coordinates scheduling. Because we receive far more inquiries than we have patient slots, our secretary gathers data regarding the referral source and presenting complaint. Prospective patients are then pre-screened for suitability by a PCAAD faculty member. Children whose presenting complaint is another disorder such as ADHD or who have been referred for a psychopharmacology evaluation are referred to associated programs within the subspecialty clinic framework. Patients who are accepted in our clinic are then scheduled for an intake evaluation.

## Preevaluation

To speed and focus the evaluation process, we gather a sizable amount of data prior to the patient's initial visit, using the same evaluation for every child seen in the subspecialty clinic. In addition to requesting psychiatric/psychological, neuropsychological, hospitalization, and school records, we ask patients and family members to complete a packet of materials designed to assess important domains of psychopathology in the context of the patient's presenting concerns. Included with the material sent in advance is a brochure describing PCAAD, our fee schedule, information about the first appointment, and a map to our office. Parents are asked to mail the questionnaires back to us before the initial visit and are informed that the patient will not be seen if the material is not completed.

Table 2.2 summarizes the information elicited by the Conners–March Developmental Questionnaire (Conners & March, 1996). Table 2.3 lists the rating scales we typically ask the child and parent to complete. Some of these scales, such as the Multidimensional Anxiety Scale for Children (MASC) and the Child and Adolescent Trauma Survey (CATS), are research scales that will soon be released for

---

**TABLE 2.2.** Information Elicited by the Conners–March Developmental Questionnaire (Conners & March, 1996)

Demographics
History of presenting problem
Previous treatment providers
Medication history
Birth and pregnancy history
Early developmental history
School history/learning problems
Peer relationships
Family psychiatric history
Family medical history
Patient medical history

**TABLE 2.3.** Rating Scales

Conners Parent Rating Scale (CPRS-R)
Conners Teacher Rating Scale (CTRS-R)
Multidimensional Anxiety Scale for Children
  (MASC)
Children's Depression Inventory (CDI)
Child and Adolescent Trauma Survey (CATS)
Leyton Obsessional Inventory

clinical use through MultiHealth Systems (MHS) in Toronto, Ontario, Canada.* Others, such as the Children's Depression Inventory and the Conners Parent and Teacher Rating Scales are already available commercially from MHS (Conners, 1995).

By gathering such data before seeing the patient, the assessing clinician is able to adjust his or her "prior probabilities" relative to the diagnosis of OCD and estimate the likelihood of complicating comorbidities. Stated differently, if you know a great deal about the patient from the use of rating scale and other data, it is much easier to focus quickly on the primary problem(s) besetting the child and family. Even better, it is also possible to move quickly past the level of diagnosis to individual symptoms by looking at rating scales from the perspective of individual items. For example, a child might display contamination fears (seen directly on the Leyton) and panic-level anxiety (seen on the MASC generally as fear/avoidance items and, specifically, as suffocation anxiety). In this way, it is relatively straightforward to focus on the primary and differential diagnoses, employing a "medical model" in which patients are seen as "okay" and psychiatric illness is framed as the object of treatment.

## First Appointment

The initial visit involves an extensive evaluation (lasting 1½ hours) by a child psychiatrist or psychologist. This evaluation includes a clinical interview with the child and parents covering Axis I through V of DSM-IV; careful consideration of the data from the rating scales

---

*For further information on these and other useful rating scales, contact MultiHealth Systems in Toronto, Ontario, Canada, at 1-800-456-3003.

completed before the visit, the Conners–March Developmental Questionnaire, school records, and previous mental health treatment records; a formal mental status examination; and in some cases, a specialized neurodevelopmental evaluation. Patients with OCD are evaluated using the Symptom Checklist from the YBOCS (Goodman, Price, Rasmussen, Mazure, Delgado, et al., 1989), and are assigned a baseline score on the YBOCS and the NIMH Global OC Scale (Goodman, Rasmussen, Foa, & Price, 1994).

Ideally, a structured interview, such as the Anxiety Disorders Interview Schedule for Children (ADIS; Silverman & Eisen, 1992), should be part of every diagnostic assessment. Unfortunately, we currently lack the staffing resources to complete an ADIS, which requires lengthy separate interviews of the child and one parent. Since we routinely use the ADIS with children enrolled in formal research protocols, however, we feel fairly confident that we cover all the major domains of psychopathology in the clinical interview, especially since data from the rating scales is available to confirm the findings of the clinical interview.

## MEASURES USED IN THE INITIAL ASSESSMENT OF OCD

Perhaps because of its characteristically stereotypic presentation, there is relatively little controversy concerning the general features that must be present to diagnose OCD. However, since there is substantial variation in how symptoms may present in different individuals, scales designed to assess OCD symptoms must take into consideration a wide range of symptoms.

The only currently available self-report instrument for assessing OCD in children and adolescents is the "epidemiological version" of the Leyton Obsessional Inventory—Child Version (Berg, Whitaker, Davies, Flament, & Rapoport, 1988), which we use as a screening tool in our initial evaluation. In a county-wide survey of high school students, these authors reported norms for the 20-item Leyton that showed high internal consistency and greater symptomatology in female than male respondents. Four factors were identified: general obsessive, dirt–contamination, numbers–luck, and school-related symptoms (Berg et al., 1988). Flament et al. (1988) evaluated the efficiency of the survey form of the Leyton in identifying OCD and found acceptable sensitivity (high true positive rate) and poor specificity (high false positive rate). The survey form of the Leyton is included in Appendix II.

The primary instrument for assessing OCD is the YBOCS, which is also included, along with instructions, in Appendix II. The YBOCS first uses a comprehensive symptom checklist to inventory the presence of specific obsessive–compulsive symptoms and then assesses obsessions and compulsions separately with regard to the time they consume and the distress, interference, degree of resistance, and control associated with them. A children's version, the CYBOCS, is available (Scahill et al., 1997) that mitigates the necessity of translating items related to adult contexts (e.g., work) into child contexts (e.g., school). The YBOCS has been used as a measure of change in pharmacological (DeVeaugh-Geiss et al., 1992; Riddle et al., 1992) and cognitive-behavioral (March et al., 1994) treatment studies, as well as in studies of OCD phenomenology (Rettew et al., 1992). Since the YBOCS is an interviewer-administered and rated scale, more akin to a semistructured interview, it is not suitable for self-report, although preliminary attempts have been made to generate computer (Lee Baer, personal communication, 1996) and self-report (Warren, Zgourides, & Monto, 1993) versions.

## FEEDBACK AND TREATMENT PLANNING

Toward the end of the initial visit, the patient and parents discuss the results of the evaluation with the therapist and decide on a treatment plan. During this feedback portion of the visit, the child's presenting problems are summarized in terms of DSM-IV diagnoses, which are linked to a neurodevelopmental model of OCD and to reinforcing environmental factors. After a careful discussion of our diagnostic impressions, we then make recommendations for: (1) additional assessment procedures, if required; (2) cognitive-behavioral psychotherapies; (3) pharmacotherapies; and (4), behavioral and/or pedagogic academic interventions, if required.

A typical treatment plan for an 11-year-old girl with OCD that is complicated by a possible nonverbal learning disability and by social phobia and who is from a supportive family might look like this:

- *Assessment:* Referral to a neuropsychologist for psychoeducational testing to rule out a nonverbal learning disability. PANDAS screening (nose and throat strep cultures), an ASO titer, and an anti-DNAse (strep) b antibody test to exclude pediatric autoimmune disorder associated with streptococcal infection.

• *Cognitive-behavioral psychotherapies*: To treat OCD, our OCD protocol; to treat social phobia, a developmentally sensitive implementation of the social phobia/panic protocol developed by Barlow and colleagues (Barlow & Craske, 1989) incorporated within the framework of our OCD protocol. Refer patient and family to the OC Foundation and to our local OCD support group. Provide reading list for anxiety disorders and nonverbal learning disability (NVLD).

• *Pharmacotherapy*: If CBT shows little or no benefit after 6 weeks, begin a trial of an ascending dose of a selective serotonin reuptake inhibitor, such as fluvoxamine. If anxiety is a significant barrier to successful exposure/response prevention (E/RP), consider adding a low-dose anxiolytic, such as clonazepam.

• *Academic*: Include school-based behavioral interventions for OCD as necessary; defer pedagogic interventions for NVLD pending results from the psychoeducational evaluation. Give parents a copy of an article on OCD in the school setting (e.g., Adams et al., 1994) to help them inform school personnel about OCD.

Treatment often founders because of an insufficient appreciation of Lyall's fundamental observation: "The most important leg of a three-legged stool is the one that's missing." However, this method of developing and specifying treatment is sufficiently detailed so that it is unlikely that a major treatment target has been omitted.

## SUMMARY

In assessing and planning treatment for OCD, we attempt to implement interventions that present a logically consistent and compelling relationship between the disorder, the treatment, and the specified outcome. In particular, we attempt to keep the various treatment targets distinct with respect to the various treatment interventions so that aspects of the symptom picture that are likely to respond to a psychosocial rather than a psychopharmacological intervention are kept as distinct as possible. This method allows us to review in detail the indications, risks, and benefits of proposed and alternative treatments with parents and patient in a detailed way. After this discussion, parents and patient generally choose a treatment protocol consisting of CBT alone or CBT in combination with an appropriate medication intervention.

# Chapter 3

## Overview of Treatment

He has not learned the lesson of life who does not every day
surmount a fear.
—*Ralph Waldo Emerson*, Society and Solitude,
*"Courage"* (1870)

In this chapter, we first describe the theoretical foundations that
inform the cognitive-behavioral treatment of pediatric OCD. In doing
so, we present a dictionary of terms that are commonplace among
therapists who apply CBT to the various pediatric anxiety disorders.
For readers familiar with social learning theory, our descriptions will
be straightforward, perhaps even a bit simplistic. For those not familiar
with the theory and terminology of CBT, reading these sections
carefully will yield dividends when you find yourself teaching these
same concepts to your patients. After defining the terminology, we
then provide an overview of the treatment protocol itself before
concluding this chapter with a discussion of logistical and other issues
that influence the implementation of treatment.

### THEORETICAL FOUNDATIONS

This CBT program falls theoretically within the framework of social
learning theory, in which both behavioral and cognitive information

processing approaches to modifying symptoms are emphasized (Foa & Kozak, 1985). In particular, behavioral psychotherapists work with patients to change behaviors and thereby to reduce distressing thoughts and feelings. Cognitive therapists work to first change thoughts and feelings, with improvements in functional behavior following in turn. Our program uses both cognitive and behavioral interventions, and so falls within the purview of CBT. Like pharmacotherapy, which seeks to modify thoughts, feelings, and behaviors by directly manipulating the functional neuroanatomy that mediates these effects, CBT also can be seen as an effective method for returning aberrant central nervous system information processing to a more normal state (Schwartz, 1996).

## VOCABULARY BUILDING

Like most theoretically derived treatments, CBT has its own vocabulary. Although it isn't necessary to be expert in applied behavioral analysis to work effectively with youngsters with OCD, it is important to master the concepts that underlie the treatment interventions effective for OCD and other anxiety disorders. In Table 3.1, we list some of the more important terms you will need to know with their definitions and examples of their implementation. If you spend a few minutes carefully perusing this table, it will make it easier to move through other sections of this book. Familiarity with the concepts behind the terms is essential to teaching these concepts, if not the terminology itself, to your patients.

## THERAPY PROCESS VARIABLES

While the basic exposure plus response prevention (E/RP) paradigm is the same for youth and adults, there are clear differences in the processes of therapy between children and adults that spell the difference between success and failure in treatment. While developing this treatment protocol, we necessarily identified several important therapeutic nuances that serve to decrease resistance to CBT and to increase the probability that E/RP will be successful. What are these therapy process variables, and how do they differ between pediatric

**TABLE 3.1.** Definition of Terms

| Term | Definition | Examples |
| --- | --- | --- |
| Cognitive-behavioral therapy (CBT) | CBT provides cognitive and behavioral corrective information that targets specific symptoms in a way that logically connects theory, interventions, and outcome. | Behavioral psychotherapy for anxiety disorders (emphasizing fear reduction), for depression (emphasizing improvement in affect, relationships and decreases in depressogenic cognitions), and for disruptive behaviors (emphasizing clear communication and rewards and consequences). |
| Obsession | Intrusive thoughts, urges, images, or ideas characteristic of OCD, usually accompanied by a dysphoric affect (e.g., doubt, feeling of incompleteness, anxiety, disgust, or aggressive feelings or urges). | Contamination fears. |
| Compulsion | An intentional behavior, often performed in a stereotyped or ritualized fashion, designed to reduce an obsession and accompanying dysphoric affects. | Washing or checking rituals. |
| Mental ritual | A compulsion that is done using thoughts only. | Praying to cancel out a "sinful" thought. |
| Exposure | The exposure principle states that anxiety will decrease after prolonged contact with the phobic stimulus in the absence of real threat. | For example, a patient with fear of heights goes up a ladder: the first time it is scary; the tenth time it is boring. |
| Contrived exposure | Exposure in which the patient seeks out and confronts anxiety-provoking situations or triggers. | Intentionally touching a "contaminated" toilet seat. |
| Uncontrived exposure | Exposure to phobic stimuli that cannot easily be avoided during routine daily activities. | Touching the toilet seat because you have to use the restroom in the course of daily living. |
| Avoidance | Purposeful attempt not to encounter phobic stimuli in order to reduce anxiety. | Refusal to use a public restroom because of contamination fears. |

*(cont.)*

**TABLE 3.1** (*cont.*)

| Term | Definition | Examples |
|------|-----------|----------|
| Escape–avoidance | After encountering a phobic stimulus, fleeing before habituation has a chance to occur; escape–avoidance dramatically reinforces anxiety and reduces future compliance with CBT. | During a contrived exposure task, say touching a toilet seat, leaving to do a ritual, say washing hands, before anxiety returns to zero. |
| Response prevention | The response prevention principle states that adequate exposure is only possible in the absence of rituals or compulsions. | Not doing the ritual—for example, washing—after either contrived or uncontrived exposure—for example, touching a toilet seat. |
| Exposure plus response prevention (E/RP) | Contrived or uncontrived exposure plus refraining from performing compulsions. | Seeking out a toilet seat, touching it, and then *not* washing hands. |
| Imaginal exposure | Exposure (and response prevention) performed in imagination rather than in vivo. Imaginal exposure is usually lower on the hierarchy than in vivo exposure and serves as an easier rehearsal for in vivo exposure. Also, since a patient's OCD triggers may not be available in the office setting, imaginal exposure may be the only method by which the therapist and patient can approach a specific OCD target symptom. | Touching a toilet seat and not washing in imagination. |
| Habituation | A neurobehavioral response in which symptoms decrease across successive exposure trials. | Decreased anxiety about contamination with repeated E/RP directed to contamination triggers. |
| Positive reinforcement | Imposition of a pleasurable stimulus to increase a desirable behavior. | Praise after successfully resisting OCD. |
| Punishment | Imposition of an aversive stimulus to decrease an undesirable behavior. Punishment increases anxiety and decreases motivation to resist OCD. | "Grounding" because of OCD symptoms. |

**TABLE 3.1** (*cont.*)

| Term | Definition | Examples |
|------|-----------|----------|
| Negative reinforcement | Self-reinforcing purposeful removal of an aversive stimulus. Or, stated differently, the termination of an aversive stimulus, which when stopped, increases or stamps in the behavior that removed the aversive stimulus. | Scratching an itch is a classic negative reinforcement paradigm. Compulsions provide short-term relief of obsessional anxiety via negative reinforcement, while reinforcing OCD over the long haul. In a sense, OCD itself can be seen as a tonic aversive stimulus. Looked at this way, the increase in enthusiasm for treatment that accompanies successful CBT works in part because of negative reinforcement (e.g., treatment-induced reduction in OCD symptoms increases compliance with CBT). |
| Extinction | Because blocking rituals or avoidance behaviors removes the negative reinforcement effect of the rituals or avoidance, response prevention technically is an extinction procedure. By convention, however, extinction is usually defined as the elimination of OCD-related behaviors through removal of parental positive reinforcement. | Refusal to reassure the anxious patient. |
| Subjective units of discomfort (SUDS) | Extent of distress when doing a contrived or uncontrived exposure task rated on an interval scale from 1 to 10. | Using a fear thermometer to determine the level of dysphoric affect associated with presentation of a phobic stimulus in the absence of anxiety-reducing rituals. |
| Stimulus hierarchy | A list of phobic stimuli ranked from least to most difficult to resist using SUDS scores. | Unique list of OCD specific contamination fears ranked by SUDS score. An individual patient may have one or more hierarchies, depending on the complexity of OCD. For example, a particular patient may have separate hierarchies for contamination fears and for repeating rituals. |

(*cont.*)

**TABLE 3.1** (*cont.*)

| Term | Definition | Examples |
| --- | --- | --- |
| Transition/ work zone | Items on the stimulus hierarchy where the patient is successful at resisting OCD at least one-third of the time. The transition/work zone provides a reliable guide to selecting E/RP targets that match the child's ability to resist OCD successfully. | E/RP targets at the lower end of the stimulus hierarchy. |
| Flooding versus graded E/RP | Graded exposure begins low on the hierarchy; flooding begins with the most difficult items. | Children generally do not tolerate flooding, which unwitting results when the therapist specifies an E/RP procedure that is too difficult. Allowing the child to choose E/RP targets from the transition/work zone minimizes this risk. |
| Differential reinforcement of other behavior (DRO) | For example, parental attention directed toward mutually pleasant interactions and away from potentially negative interactions, as in playing games while not commenting on OCD rituals. | Playing checkers while waiting for anxiety to decrease during E/RP. Refraining from giving advice. |
| Generalization training | Moving the methods and success of E/RP to targets not specifically addressed on the stimulus hierarchy. | E/RP for all toilets/sinks in the universe. |
| Relapse prevention | Interventions designed to anticipate triggers for reemergence of OCD symptoms; practicing CBT skillful coping in advance. | Imaginal exposure to a contamination fear followed by using CT and RP to successfully resist the incursion of OCD. |

patients and adults? In general, they are means by which the therapist ensures that everyone is allied on the side of the child in the contest with OCD, and through which the therapist teaches a strategy that enables the child to master E/RP tasks. Specific therapy process variables that form recurring themes in the treatment of pediatric OCD include the following.

## Externalizing OCD

One key to establishing a successful therapeutic alliance is to clearly separate OCD from the child and family, a process termed "externalizing the problem" by the Australian family therapist, Michael White. Borrowing from White's narrative therapy techniques (White, 1986; White & Epston, 1990), we describe OCD as an unpleasant and oppressive neurobehavioral illness over which both child and family already have some influence—an influence we and they desire to increase. In this way, therapist, child, and family become members of the same team with a unified goal of helping the child get OCD out of her life.

## Gradual versus Intensive Exposure

Anxious youngsters typically like treatment to be predictable and controllable. Graded exposure involves weekly sessions in which the child has explicit control over selection of exposure targets, which are then primarily addressed through homework assignments. This form of gradual exposure provides a greater degree of control than intensive exposure, which relies on daily sessions using therapist-assisted E/RP. Since young persons tolerate anxiety less well than most adults, it helps to make the treatment predictable, controllable, and most importantly, successful. Thus, graded exposure is probably better for most children and adolescents, though some prefer and others require intensive exposure to make progress against OCD. For example, some adolescents who have been battling OCD for years need to be encouraged to consider choosing higher level exposure tasks early on so that their motivation for treatment can be stimulated by seeing improvement more quickly.

## Therapist versus Patient Control

The whole idea of behavior therapy often brings to mind a strong-willed therapist telling the patient what to do. Since most children already know that OCD is senseless, this usually sounds to the child like "just stop that bad habit and you'll be fine." Additionally, because children typically don't tolerate anxiety as well as adults, having the therapist choose E/RP targets presents a greater risk of inadvertently turning graded exposure into flooding, which reduces compliance with treatment. It is crucial that the treatment not appear as punishment to the child. We therefore recommend telling the children up front that we won't ask them to do anything that they're not ready for, and that the choice of E/RP targets is theirs to make. We simply insist on progress, not on a set rate of progress.

To facilitate the choice of E/RP targets, we use the concept of the "transition or work zone." Borrowing from Michael White again, we first look for situations in which the child is successful in resisting OCD some of the time. For example, the therapist might ask, "Give me an example of a time in the last week when you didn't let OCD boss you around." Using these exceptions to the rule that OCD always wins, the patient then clearly spells out a region on the stimulus hierarchy in which he or she wins sometimes and loses sometimes. This region is then labeled the transition or work zone, because (1) it defines the transition between territory controlled by the child and territory controlled by OCD, and (2) it is where the child will work to boss back OCD by selecting E/RP tasks. The concept is simple: It is more likely that the child will be successful at E/RP if she chooses to try to become 100% successful at an E/RP task at which she is already partially successful than if the therapist chooses E/RP tasks on a hit or miss basis.

Therapists may find that the term "transition zone," a carto-graphic metaphor used to show the boundary between OCD and the child's life space graphically, is more effective in explaining these concepts to some children (see Handout 2, Appendix I). For children who need a more concrete and direct approach, an alternative term— the work zone—may better increase compliance with treatment. The transition zone concept helps with selection of E/RP targets by defin-ing a "win some, lose some" region that can be converted to "win all the time" with the implementation of E/RP. After E/RP targets are selected, the therapist can present the idea of doing E/RP tasks chosen from the transition/work zone as analogous to other work the child does on a regular basis, such as chores or homework. As with other chores, E/RP tasks chosen from the work zone require commitment and effort on the part of the child, and may to some extent get in the way of other, often more pleasant, activities. In this regard, the work zone approach communicates an expectation that the child must do the work to get better—just as he must practice the guitar to become proficient as a guitarist—and also reinforces the idea that the therapist as coach is responsible for the structure of the treatment while the initiative for change is left to the child. For some children who are reluctant to participate fully in E/RP because it is a boring chore, rather than out of avoidance, increasing the density of reinforcement (as in behavioral contracting) may be very helpful in improving commitment to treatment. For such children, the work zone concept is often more beneficial than relying on intrinsic motivation to be rid of OCD as embodied in the concept of the transition zone. For most, if not all, children, both concepts are often helpful at different times in treatment. For example, the transition zone concept works well at the start when the youngster is worried about E/RP and needs the therapist to maximize the predictability and controllability of the treatment; later, when the child is slowly moving up the upper part of the stimulus hierarchy, the work zone concept may be a better metaphor since treatment at this point realistically feels like hard work. Finally, these two concepts are often helpful in communicating to parents the difference between *can't* (some things lie outside the transition zone) and *won't* (the child just didn't commit to doing the homework). Such clarification makes it easier for parents to know how much to comfort and how much to push the child with respect to compliance with E/RP.

## Therapist-Assisted E/RP versus OCD Homework

OCD typically involves many triggers that are located at some distance from the therapist's office. Going to a patient's home or work situation can be very helpful, especially in intensive treatment protocols in which the therapist assumes more initiative in forcing E/RP (Foa & Wilson, 1991); however, this usually isn't very practical with young patients. Since we use a graded office-based E/RP model, we rehearse in vivo homework using office-based imaginal exposure, and where possible, office-based E/RP, recruiting parents and other sympathetic individuals to provide assistance at home. Occasionally, when moving to a more intensive model because of difficult-to-manage OCD, we go outside the office setting to provide in vivo therapist-assisted E/RP.

## Developmental Considerations

It goes without saying that it is crucial to adjust the treatment so that it is appropriate to each patient's level of cognitive functioning, social maturity, and capacity for sustained attention. As noted in Chapter 1, developmental considerations may interact with the diagnosis of OCD: bedtime rituals, eating or dressing rituals, and making collections of objects are common in children at different ages. Younger patients require more redirection and activities; adolescents are more sensitive to the effects of OCD on peer interactions, which in turn requires more discussion. Cognitive interventions, especially, need to be adjusted to the developmental level of the patient. For example, adolescents are typically less likely than younger children to appreciate giving OCD a "nasty nickname." Developmental themes involving separation (becoming your own boss) and individuation (becoming your own person) may affect your ability to implement treatment. For example, children who are grappling with separation–individuation themes may find that OCD is tangled up in "boss battles," which are inherently developmental in nature, and may consequently have some difficulty engaging in CBT. Such difficulties may be more common in the early elementary years and in early adolescence. In contrast, children in middle childhood, who are in what Erik Erikson labeled the industry versus inferiority phase, may do better with E/RP; for these children, the effort involved in E/RP itself is rewarding not only because they are beating OCD but also because it contributes to their sense of industry and, therefore, the resulting anxiety cost is "worth it." In either case, helping the child and parents differentiate what is developmental and what is related to OCD, and how the two interact, will help move the therapist, patient, and family toward a treatment plan they can all agree on.

## Graded Family Involvement

Each family is different, so that treatment must be individualized with respect to the extent of family involvement. As discussed in Chapter 19, which addresses working with families, we grade family involvement as a function of the extent to which (1) family members are tangled up by OCD or (2) family problems interfere with the treatment of OCD. Too little family involvement may reduce the effectiveness of CBT; too much involvement and therapy may not only stall, but may also (appropriately) make the family angry. In all cases, we provide family members with extensive information about OCD and its treatment and help them to ally with the affected child in the struggle with OCD. To get treatment started on the best possible footing, during the first treatment session, we instruct parents in two specific interventions, "stop giving advice" and differential reinforcement of other behavior (DRO), which are also provided as homework for the first treatment session.

## Stylistic Considerations

Many therapists are accustomed to empathic nondirective listening and, especially, to play therapy techniques. While good listening skills and creative play are important to CBT, play therapy per se works poorly for the cognitive-behavioral psychotherapist who needs to actively structure treatment interventions. For example, cognitive-behavioral therapists usually ask question after question designed to elicit details about how OCD oppresses the patient and how the patient successfully resists OCD (e.g., "Can you be more specific?"; "Tell me more about that."; "Can you give me an example of what we're talking about from the last week or so?") Other stylistic considerations, such as greater self-disclosure, modeling risk taking, and extensive use of humor, are also important to successful CBT.

## SUMMARY OF THE TREATMENT PROTOCOL

Table 3.2 summarizes the treatment protocol. It is assumed that the child has already completed a thorough evaluation. Treatment takes place in four steps usually distributed over 12 to 20 sessions. Each session includes a statement of goals, a careful review of the preceding week, introduction of new information, therapist-assisted "nuts and bolts" practice, homework for the coming week, and monitoring procedures. Information sheets describing the goals and homework for that week are given at the end of each session. Step One focuses on psychoeducation during two sessions in the first week. Step Two, cognitive training (CT) begins in the first week and continues in the second, while Step Three, mapping OCD, is completed during two sessions in the second week.

**TABLE 3.2.** CBT Treatment Protocol

| Visit number | Goals |
| --- | --- |
| Session 1 | Psychoeducation |
| Session 2 | Cognitive training (CT) |
| Session 3 | CT/mapping OCD |
| Session 4 | Further mapping |
| Weeks 3–18 | Exposure and response prevention (E/RP) |
| Weeks 18–19 | Relapse prevention |
| Sessions 1, 7, and 12 | Parent sessions |

These first three steps form the basis for Step Four, which initiates intensive graded E/RP over weeks 3–20, though many children require far fewer sessions.

In writing this manual, we have generally used the word "child" to indicate a child or adolescent. However, where special age-related issues arise, we specify younger children or adolescents. It has been our goal to use clear, nontechnical language throughout the manual so that it would be accessible to therapists from a variety of backgrounds. We encourage those using this program to broaden their knowledge of the disorder by reading many other books on OCD treatment. We have provided tips and clinical pearls in every chapter. Although these are generally included in the description of the phase of treatment where they seem most likely to be useful, such tips might be helpful at any point in treatment. It is therefore important that therapists carefully read the book as a whole before starting treatment.

## Step One: Psychoeducation

Step One places OCD firmly within a neurobehavioral model by linking OCD with a specific set of behavioral treatments and a desired outcome—symptom reduction. To cement the neurobehavioral framework, the therapist makes use of analogies to medical illnesses such as asthma or diabetes. Metaphors for obsessions are also introduced, with ideas such as brain hiccups or problems with the volume control knob used with younger children.

The analogy to medical illness is not as far-fetched as it might at first seem. Since OCD has its roots in disordered information processing in the brain, changes in symptoms brought about by CBT ought to reflect changes in brain function, which is just what Lew Baxter and Jeff Schwartz discovered when they looked at images of the brain at work in OCD patients before and after drug or behavior therapy. In those patients who responded to treatment, the PET images returned to normal in patients treated with drugs *and* in patients treated with CBT (Schwartz, 1996; Schwartz, Stoessel, Baxter, Martin, & Phelps, 1996). Looked at in this way, patients with OCD can be approached in the same way as patients with diabetes—only the target organ, and thus the symptom picture, differs. The treatment of each disorder involves the use of medications (e.g., insulin in diabetes, a serotonin reuptake inhibitor in OCD). In both disorders, psychosocial interventions are used to change the somatic substrate toward more normal function (e.g. diet and exercise in diabetes; CBT in OCD). Finally, not everyone gets completely well, so some interventions need to target coping with residual symptoms (e.g., diabetic foot care in diabetes; CBT, support groups, and family psychotherapy in OCD)

In addition to an extensive discussion of OCD as a medical illness, Step One also presents the risks and benefits of behavioral treatment for OCD and reviews specific details of the treatment protocol. Step One also begins the process of externalizing OCD, with younger children giving OCD a nasty nickname. By always using a disparaging name to refer to OCD, the therapist "externalizes" OCD (White, 1986) so that OCD becomes a discrete "enemy" and not a "bad habit" that may have been associated with previous punishment experiences. Adolescents frequently find this procedure silly, and prefer to refer to OCD by its medical appellation, but the principle of externalizing the disorder remains the same. Adolescents and parents ordinarily appreciate a more detailed discussion of OCD as a neurobehavioral disorder. Approaching OCD in this way allows the family and the therapist to ally with the child in order to "boss back" OCD, and thereby provides a narrative scaffolding on which to hang family interventions.

## Step Two: Cognitive Training

Step Two introduces CT, defined as training in cognitive tactics for resisting OCD (as distinct from response prevention for mental rituals). Goals of CT include increasing a sense of personal efficacy, predictability, controllability, and self-attributed likelihood of a positive outcome for E/RP tasks. Targets for CT include reinforcing accurate information regarding OCD and its treatment, cognitive resistance ("bossing back OCD"), and self-administered positive reinforcement and encouragement. To increase the patient's sense of predictability and controllability, we explicitly frame E/RP as the strategy and the therapist and parents (and sometimes teacher or friends) as the allies in the child's "battle" against OCD. Constructive self-talk ("bossing back OCD") and the use of positive coping strategies provide the child with a cognitive "tool kit" to use during exposure and response prevention tasks, which in turn facilitates E/RP compliance.

## Step Three: Mapping OCD

Step Three maps the child's experience with OCD, including specific obsessions, compulsions, triggers, avoidance behaviors, and consequences. In behavioral terms, this process generate a "stimulus

hierarchy" within a narrative context. We use cartographic metaphors, shown in Handout 2 (Appendix I), to illustrate where the
child is free from OCD, where OCD and the child each "win" some
of the time, and where the child feels helpless against OCD. We call
the central region, where the child already has some success in
resisting OCD, the transition zone. Continuing the map metaphor,
"standing" with the child on territory free from OCD allows us to
strengthen the twin beliefs that we are, first, on his or her side in
the struggle against OCD, and second, interested in him or her as a
person who wants desperately to write OCD out of the story. In one
of the clinical pearls that drives the treatment forward, the therapist
teaches the child to recognize and use the transition zone, thereby
providing a reliable guide to graded exposure throughout the treatment program. In practice, the transition zone is usually defined by
the lower end of the stimulus hierarchy. As mentioned earlier, the
transition zone can also be called the work zone.

Steps Two and Three include easy trial E/RP tasks to gauge the
patient's tolerance of anxiety, level of understanding, and willingness
or ability to comply with treatment. At the same time, these tasks
instill the idea that it is possible to successfully resist and ultimately
"win" against OCD. Trial E/RP tasks also indicate whether the transition zone has been accurately located, thereby avoiding disruptive
"surprises" due to mistargeted goals for exposure or response prevention.

## Step Four: Graded Exposure and Response Prevention

Step Four fully implements the core of CBT for anxiety disorders,
namely, graded E/RP, including therapist-assisted imaginal and in vivo
E/RP practice linked to weekly homework assignments. "Exposure"
occurs when children expose themselves to the feared object, action,
or thought. "Response prevention" is the process of blocking rituals
and/or minimizing avoidance behaviors. Take, for example, the child
with a contamination fear about touching door knobs. In this case,
since door knobs trigger the obsession, the exposure task would require
the child to touch the "contaminated" door knob until his or her
anxiety disappears. Response prevention takes place when the child
refuses to perform the usual anxiety-driven compulsion, such as washing hands or using a tissue to grasp the door knob.

As in a contest, OCD is framed as the adversary, and all parties
remain intransigent against OCD. This attitude explicitly requires that

the child use his allies (the therapist and parents or friends) and new strategies (CT and E/RP) to resist OCD, thereby preventing the therapy from becoming an excuse to avoid exposure. However, since only the child can do the actual combat (the E/RP), he or she necessarily remains in charge of choosing targets from the transition or work zone. We update the transition/work zone at the beginning of each session as the child becomes more competent and successful at resisting OCD.

## The Role of Parents

Beginning with Step One, which emphasizes psychoeducation, parents are an important part of the treatment process. Parents are explicitly included in Sessions 1, 7, 12, and 19. At the end of Step One, parents receive an information booklet ("Tips for Parents," included in Appendix III) that includes tips for handling OCD. Parents check in with the therapist at the beginning and/or end of each session and we invite parents to comment on how the child is progressing in the struggle against OCD. Parent Sessions 7 and 12 focus on incorporating targets for parental response prevention or extinction, with the child again selecting targets from the transition/work zone. Session 19 focuses on generalization training and relapse prevention.

Homework assignments are presented each week with individualized clues to help the child successfully "boss back" OCD. We use positive reinforcers liberally (e.g., within-session praise and small goodies, such as pencils or gum, and between-session larger rewards, such as a trip for pizza with friends). In order to facilitate positive reinforcement and extinguish punishment by adults and peers, we also make a special effort to help youngsters tell other people (such as friends, teachers, or grandparents) how they have successfully reduced OCD's influence over their lives.

Treatment ends with a graduation ceremony, followed by a booster session 6 weeks later.

## LOGISTICAL CONSIDERATIONS

### Frequency and Number of Sessions

Questions about the frequency and number of sessions are often uppermost in the minds of children and parents. The first four sessions, which mainly involve teaching and information gathering, can be scheduled twice weekly, and it is best to schedule these initial sessions no more than a week apart. In addition to building rapport and enlisting the child's cooperation in the treatment process, these first few sessions lay the groundwork for teaching the child to think differently about OCD. It is also important to explain the treatment process early on to both children and adolescents, with particular emphasis on the centrality of exposure and response prevention. Beginning with Session 5, sessions can be scheduled at weekly or, if necessary, biweekly intervals. If biweekly sessions are necessary, we recommend using phone calls between sessions to adjust E/RP procedures.

## Location of Sessions

Where should CBT sessions be held? The therapist need not be bound to the office, although often that is the case out of necessity. When the bulk of the session involves E/RP practice, field trips to places that will trigger OCD are especially valuable. The therapist should also develop creative ways to practice E/RP in the office (e.g., bringing in household items, such as a chemical cleanser, to serve as a trigger for E/RP practice).

## Length of Sessions

How long should sessions last and how should they be organized? The usual format of sessions is shown in Table 3.3. Each session in our program lasts approximately 50 to 60 minutes. Before the session begins, parents are given a handout of parent tips for the week and encouraged to read these while the child is in with the therapist and jot down any questions they may want to ask during the 10-minute

**TABLE 3.3.** Structure of Treatment Sessions

| Session goals | Time |
| --- | --- |
| Check in with child and parents | 5 minutes |
| Review homework | 5 minutes |
| Teaching/learning tasks for week | 20 minutes |
| Discuss and agree on homework | 10 minutes |
| Parent review of session and homework | 10 minutes |

parent check-in at the end of the session. This procedure can be modified for adolescents who come alone, by giving parents tips for Sessions 1–4 during the first session.

The first 10 minutes of each session are spent checking in with the child and reviewing the previous week's homework. If the child was unable to complete the homework, this time is spent identifying what obstacles interfered with its completion.

The next 20 minutes are spent presenting the goals for the current session followed by E/RP practice. As treatment progresses, 30–40 minutes of each session may be spent in therapist-assisted exposure tasks.

Before assigning homework, a few minutes are spent obtaining ratings on the NIMH Global OC Scale and the Clinical Global Impairment and Improvement (CGI) Scales (see Appendix II). This evaluation usually goes very quickly once the child learns the rating scales. We usually obtain ratings on the YBOCS at baseline, every 3–4 weeks during treatment, and at the end of treatment. We usually graph the results of these assessments, since watching the scores come down can be one of the most rewarding parts of the treatment sessions.

The final 10 minutes are spent helping the child choose the week's homework task and reviewing strategies to increase homework success.

A brief check-in with the parent is done at the end of the session to answer any immediate questions or concerns.

As a reward for participating in the hard work of E/RP, time at the end of the session may also be allocated to a social reward (e.g., playing a game or talking about something besides OCD).

## Using the Telephone

Every child in our clinic is given our home and work telephone numbers. Some of our patients also communicate with us via email. Midweek phone calls are particularly valuable because they allow the therapist to check on how E/RP practice is going and to troubleshoot problems (e.g., poor compliance; mistargeted E/RP) that come up between sessions. For example, an E/RP task that is too difficult often causes the child to bail out of the exposure and do the compulsion anyway; this in turn reinforces OCD. Delaying compulsions is helpful *only* if the compulsion never takes place. If the exposure task is too difficult, or too easy, a new target with a greater chance of success can be chosen over the telephone. At the beginning of treatment, we schedule telephone follow-up; as treatment progresses, the children and parents know that they can call whenever necessary.

## More on Stylistic Considerations

Some therapists prefer to be nondirective and let the child's internal processes emerge naturally; others are more directive and include lots of therapist activity during the session. While the former often gravitate toward psychodynamic "play therapy" techniques and the later toward CBT or family therapy, it is important to note that therapists of all persuasions can effectively use this protocol if they follow the methods outlined here. Therapists may, of course, need to adjust their habitual style of therapy to fit the treatment of OCD. Failure to do so will be frustrating to therapist and patient and should prompt therapists to consider whether CBT is something they are suited to undertake. If the answer is "no," referral to another provider who is expert in the CBT of OCD is the treatment of choice. If the answer is "yes," all the skills that enable expert clinicians to work effectively with patients and families can be applied in using CBT to help children cope skillfully with OCD.

CBT for OCD may at first feel counterintuitive since the therapist assists the child to "choose to be anxious" rather than providing reassurance, counterarguments, or distractions to reduce such anxiety. It is vital that therapists remain on the side of the child, not OCD, even when the child encourages the opposite. The therapist may be tempted to provide unnecessary reassurance or to try to understand "why" the child has OCD, but this will not be helpful for the child. In addition, the role of "therapist as coach" emphasizes that the real therapeutic work takes place in the framework of the child practicing what is learned in treatment (i.e., the therapist coaches the child once a week, but the child must practice every day in order to get better). Treatment also enhances the child's self-esteem since it emphasizes his or her increasing competence in preference to the intrusiveness of OCD or the excellence of the therapist. By assuming a consistently matter-of-fact stance, the therapist models for the child that, although anxiety can be quite uncomfortable at times, it can be tolerated and will eventually go away.

Because CBT is in some ways similar to coaching an athletic team (i.e., the coach instructs, models, insists on practice, and finally stands on the sidelines while the players play the game for keeps), it is not surprising that cognitive-behavioral therapists do a lot of active communicating, talking as well as listening. CBT requires a molecular understanding of specific symptoms, their triggers and nature, and how the patient copes successfully or unsuccessfully with them. In order to obtain this information, and work with the patient to set up an equally specific treatment intervention, therapists often need to use a Socratic dialogue in which they pepper the patient with questions about his or her experiences "bossing or being bossed around" by OCD. The therapist typically asks for more details about how the child has successfully (or unsuccessfully) resisted OCD, usually by asking for specific examples. This approach sometimes seems like a videotape replay in which the therapist and patient engage in a playful two-way interchange about the details of the child's contest with OCD.

It is crucial that the therapist keep the tone of the session friendly and focus on OCD as the adversary, so that the patient perceives both intellectually and emotionally that the therapist is his or her ally in the struggle to put an end to OCD. Using humor can be very helpful in decreasing the intensity of anxiety and increasing motivation; however, it is important to remember to poke fun *at* OCD and not the child. Examples from the therapist's varied experiences working with other patients with OCD can often help smooth the passage through choppy waters in treatment (e.g., in encouraging patients to disclose aggressive or religious obsessions or their fear of shaking hands with someone who has AIDS). Similarly, some degree of self-disclosure by the therapist is essential to the successful conduct of treatment.

## Dealing with Real Life

Although the treatment protocol specifies the format of each session, it is often easy to become sidetracked by a myriad of other "issues." For example, virtually all children and parents come into conflict over home rules to some extent. While such struggles with parents or peers may be indirectly related to OCD, they are not the focus of treatment. It is important to keep such issues separate when possible, especially since these problems would not have led the family to seek mental health care. While oppositional behavior, poor school performance, and depression can be externalized and addressed in treatment, these secondary symptoms often remit once a child has experienced some success in "bossing back" OCD. Comorbid psychiatric symptoms can also exist independently from the OCD. Unless these symptoms are interfering with the treatment of OCD, it is best to tackle OCD first, and then address the other symptoms that remain if the child and parents wish to do so. Therapists who allows other issues to sidetrack the treatment may find themselves in a maze of confusion that actually undermines the effectiveness of CBT for OCD. This is especially important for therapists with less experience with CBT for OCD, who often end up focusing on family issues or other seemingly urgent concerns rather than tackling OCD. While the therapist and patient may in the short run feel less anxious by avoiding OCD—the therapist because family issues are familiar territory; the patient because talking about something other than OCD avoids E/RP—the end result will be a decided lack of progress in reducing the impact that OCD has on the child's life.

On the other hand, while it is important to avoid getting sidetracked, it is also important to be flexible. Each child is unique; when an intervention or exposure task is not working, revision is needed. Flexibility is especially important in deciding on exposure tasks, since the child may wish to pick something too easy or, not uncommonly, too hard, or may even insist that anything and everything is impossible. A child who claims to be unable to touch textbooks may not be able to expose or "contaminate" herself with her math book, but may feel ready to resist washing after touching her English book. The therapist frequently needs to narrow down what defines the transition/ work zone for OCD symptoms in response to a specific trigger. This process requires extensive attention to detail and absolute confidence that the transition zone can be found if you simply look hard enough. Sometimes, when the child is upset about something that has just happened, such as a fight with a friend, it is impossible to get the child to focus on OCD. In such cases, the appropriate response is to help the child use the tools of CBT to understand and skillfully manage the crisis at hand. OCD will still be there the following week. Such flexibility not only facilitates the treatment process, but also guards the therapeutic relationship between therapist and child that helps to guide and strengthen the treatment—a relationship that should never be sacrificed in order to adhere to the written protocol.

## EVALUATION

We monitor the course and outcome of treatment using symptom hierarchies, fear thermometer ratings to assess within-exposure anxiety in response to specific targets, the YBOCS, the NIMH Global OC

Scale, and the CGI scales (see Appendix II). The NIMH Global OC Scale and the CGI scales, which take less than a minute, are filled out weekly. Since the YBOCS takes considerably longer to complete (about 10 minutes), we generally obtain it every 3–4 weeks. These assessments, when graphed, provides a valuable object lesson for the child and parent with respect to the child's progress in treatment.

The most detailed instrument for assessing the outcome of treatment is the YBOCS, which assess obsessions and compulsions separately in terms of time consumed, distress, interference, degree of resistance, and control (Goodman, Price, Rasmussen, Mazure, Delgado, et al., 1989; Goodman, Price, Rasmussen, Mazure, Fleischmann, et al., 1989). The YBOCS is a clinician-rated instrument that merges data from clinical observation with data from parent and child reports. The cutoffs that are generally used in evaluating the YBOCS scores are as follows:

- YBOCS 10–18: Mild OCD that causes distress but not necessarily dysfunction; help from others is usually not required to get through the day.
- YBOCS 18–29: Moderate OCD that causes both distress and functional impairment.
- YBOCS 30 or above: Severe OCD that causes serious functional impairment requiring significant help from others.

Our goal in treatment is to reach a score indicating a subclinical level of symptoms, which is generally considered to be in the range of 8–10 on the YBOCS. We also use the YBOCS Symptom Checklist to inventory past and present OCD symptoms, initial severity, total OCD severity, relative preponderance of obsessions and compulsions, and degree of insight.

The global measures of improvement and impairment involve clinician ratings based on a global judgment of how the child is doing relative to normal (impairment ratings) or to his or her baseline symptom level (improvement). The NIMH Global OC Scale (Goodman & Price, 1992) is a measure of illness severity rated from 1 (normal) through 12 (extremely impaired). The Clinical Global Impairment Scale, which measures the impairment associated with the disorder, ranges from 1 (normal, not at all ill) to 7 (extremely ill); the Clinical Global Improvement Scale is a measure of global improvement rated from 1 (very much improved) to 7 (very much worse) (Guy, 1976).

Why evaluate outcome? First, using the YBOCS, the clinician can update the symptom hierarchy at each session, minimizing the possibility that new or reemerging symptoms will be missed. Second, the YBOCS averages parent and child ratings, so that the clinician must address discrepant views of the child's progress where they exist. Third, the YBOCS provides a more detailed view of how the child is doing (e.g., in resisting OCD and gaining control over OCD symptoms). Thus, the YBOCS is a far richer source of information than the three global measures, which simply involve therapist ratings of general outcome. From the patient's point of view, the major advantage of measuring outcome is being able to visually track treatment progress. It is very satisfying to watching symptoms decrease over time (see Figures 3.1 and 3.2), especially when parents or teachers are frustrated at the slow pace of progress. Once the patient gets the hang of the YBOCS, it is not uncommon to see the whole evaluation procedure reduced to less than 5 minutes—1 or 2 minutes if the YBOCS is omitted—with patient and parents looking forward to seeing the results graphed at the end of each visit.

For the therapist familiar with single case experimental designs, this approach lends itself to within-subject multiple baseline design (March & Mulle, 1995). To illustrate this point, as well as to depict the usual course of treatment, we used a within-subject multiple baseline design plus global ratings across treatment weeks, to monitor the treatment of an 8-year-old girl with OCD with CBT alone (March & Mulle, 1995). As shown in Figure 3.1, 11 weeks of treatment

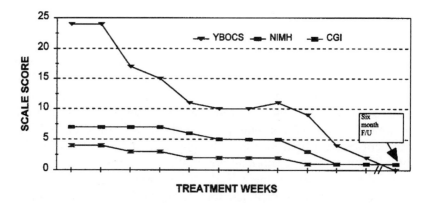

**FIGURE 3.1.** Global symptom ratings across time. From March and Mulle (1995). Copyright 1995 by Williams and Wilkins. Reprinted by permission.

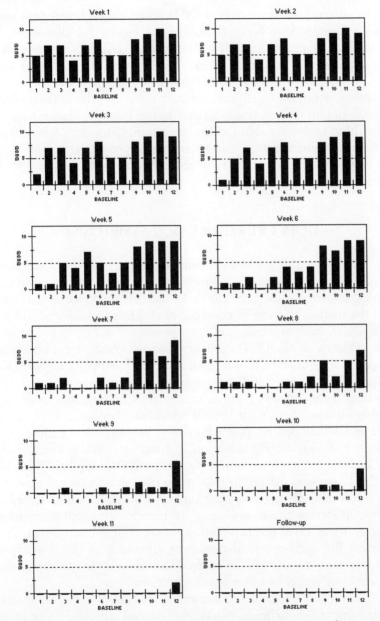

**FIGURE 3.2.** Multiple baselines over time. Symptom key: 1 = touching mouth; 2 = snack after touching plants; 3 = not washing for meals; 4 = wearing turtlenecks again; 5 = touching something sticky; 6 = touching dish liquid; 7 = use towel again; 8 = touch cat; 9 = use Ajax; 10 = use Windex; 11 = toxic paint; 12 = touching sick people. From March and Mulle (1995). Copyright 1995 by Williams and Wilkins. Reprinted by permission.

produced complete resolution of OCD symptoms and treatment gains were maintained at 6-month follow-up. Figure 3.2 illustrates the progress of treatment at each week for each baseline symptom. Each box represents a treatment week. The Y (vertical) axis represents SUDS (fear thermometer) scores for each baseline symptom on the symptom hierarchy, which are depicted as bars on the X (horizontal) axis. Symptom reduction was specific to the exposure and/or response prevention targets for that baseline symptom. Once our patient began to respond, generalization across baselines appeared, with some slowing down as she reached the most difficult symptoms at the top of the symptom hierarchy.

## DOES CBT REDUCE OCD SYMPTOMS?

We developed this treatment manual in response to deficiencies identified from a systematic literature review and from our collective clinical experience (March, 1995). In our first study, we used version 1 of the manual to treat 15 consecutive child and adolescent patients with OCD, most of whom had been previously stabilized on medications (March et al., 1994). Our child and adolescent patients, who ranged in age from 6 to 18 years old, and their families found the "How I Ran OCD Off My Land" program highly acceptable, even when it was not accompanied by rapid reduction in OCD symptoms. Statistical analyses showed significant benefit immediately posttreatment and at 6-month follow-up. At posttreatment follow-up, nine patients had achieved at least a 50% reduction in symptoms on the YBOCS and had become clinically asymptomatic on the NIMH Global OC Scale. Of the 12 patients defined as responders (i.e., those who had a greater than 30% percent improvement on the YBOCS), none relapsed at follow-up intervals over as long as 18 months, although several had brief episodes of recurrent symptoms that required additional CBT sessions. Booster behavioral treatment allowed 6 of the 9 asymptomatic patients to discontinue medication, again without relapse after 6 months or longer of follow-up observation.

Since these 15 patients represented all patients who came to us for treatment (excluding consults, hospitalized patients, those living at extended distances, and patients treated by other therapists), we concluded that our protocol-driven implementation of CBT represents a safe, effective, and acceptable treatment program for OCD in young persons. We have since completed a series of single-subject designs with much the same results (see March & Mulle, 1995). Equally important, other researchers in pediatric anxiety disorders have had similar experiences using our treatment protocol (Edna Foa, personal communication, 1996). We also often hear success stories from the more than 3,000 clinicians who have received an earlier version of the manual from us or from the OC Foundation. We therefore conclude that cognitive-behavioral psychotherapy, alone or in combination with pharmacotherapy, appears to be a safe, acceptable, and effective treatment for OCD in children and adolescents.

## WHAT'S NEXT

On the following pages, we present a session-by-session guide to the cognitive-behavioral treatment of OCD. Each session includes a statement of goals, procedures to meet those goals, and a means of evaluating the outcome. We also include tips for therapists and parents as well as guidelines for developmental considerations. Topics from the next session are always introduced at the end of the preceding session. For example, trial E/RP tasks begin almost immediately, but formal E/RP doesn't start until the transition/work zone has been carefully and clearly located and the child has his "tool kit" in place. Similarly, we anticipate involving parents at visit 7 by rehearsing parental E/RP with the child at visit 6. We have found that anticipating interventions in this way dramatically reduces anticipatory anxiety.

# Part Two

# SESSION-BY-SESSION TREATMENT PROGRAM

The guide, the therapist, will specify to the patient the action as precisely as possible. He will analyze it into its elements . . . to give the patient's mind an immediate and proximate aim. By continually repeating the order to perform the action, that is, exposure, he will help the patient greatly.

—*Pierre Janet, 1903*

Following Janet's injunction to be precise in implementing exposure-based treatment of OCD, in Chapters 4–16, we provide a session-by-session guide to the treatment of OCD. Sessions 1–4 quickly set the stage for beginning exposure and are designed to be completed in the first 2 weeks (with two sessions per week). All other sessions take place on a weekly basis.

Although we provide a great deal of information in the chapters describing the early sessions, this does not reflect the amount of time we expect the therapist to devote to each topic. However, beginning therapists tend to find the additional information, and especially the sample dialogues, helpful early in treatment, while less information is needed later as comfort with CBT increases. A similar process takes place for the patient.

We suggest that therapists first read through all the sessions quickly, and then review each session more carefully, considering how the treatment techniques might be applied to a specific child with OCD. Before beginning each session, therapists may find it helpful to review the manual and make notes if necessary to guide the progress of the session. We encourage therapists to make marginal notes detailing the "clinical pearls" they discover in treating different patients with different problems. Such hints can help you with subsequent patients.*

Although an average course of CBT is 12 to 20 sessions, which is the format we use here, the number of sessions depends on the patient's progress and, to some extent, on the therapist's familiarity with CBT for patients with OCD. Since each session builds on skills learned in the preceding session, it is better to proceed more slowly and accomplish the session goals than to skip a session in the interest of finishing sooner. Thus, although the middle E/RP sessions are tagged to specific treatment weeks, the therapist can and should expand or contract the number of sessions depending on the patient's response to treatment. Likewise, the timing of family sessions can be tailored somewhat to better reflect the grading of family targets for a particular child. In contrast, the beginning sessions, which focus on setting the framework for treatment, mapping OCD, and teaching the "tool kit" should not vary; similarly, the final sessions on relapse prevention and generalization training are necessary for all patients.

## CASE EXAMPLE

The case example we use throughout this manual to illustrate the session-by-session treatment strategies is based on a composite of many children with OCD whom we have treated. This example involves a therapist we call Nadine and her patient Carla. Nadine is a registered nurse who works in a mental health clinic. She has had supervised training in CBT and works primarily with children and adolescents

---

*Parenthetically, we are always happy to receive comments on how the treatment program might be improved. If you wish to pass on helpful hints or other comments about how the manual did or didn't work for you and your patients, please send them to us at Duke University Medical Center.

who have OCD and other pediatric anxiety disorders. Carla is an 8-year-old girl with germ worries and a need for symmetry. Carla worries about touching plants, the cat, something sticky, dishwashing liquid, toxic paint, cleaning fluids, and people who are sick. She also fears becoming sick if she does not periodically wipe her mouth with her shirt. Carla's germ worries are typically triggered on a daily basis by things such as school books, sink handles, and public restrooms. Carla responds to these germ worries by washing her hands before and after touching the contaminated object. When possible, she prefers to avoid contaminated objects or places altogether. For example, she avoids touching plants. Carla's need for symmetry manifests itself in balancing "touches and looks." If someone touches Nadine on her right arm, she must touch her left arm in the same place or, if Carla looks at one side of a hung picture, she must also look at the other side. Carla also has a need to balance her gaze when she is reading and writing, which has made it very difficult for her to complete her school assignments. Nadine and Carla appear in sample dialogues during each session in the following chapters. We hope that such clinical examples will help clinicians understand the theory and techniques that are most effective in running OCD off your patients' land.

# Chapter 4

## Session 1: Establishing a Neurobehavioral Framework

At the beginning of the first session, Nadine spends some time getting to know Carla's likes and dislikes and her special interests. She learns that Carla is an aspiring artist and likes to draw. As Nadine explains to Carla that OCD is a kind of "hiccup" in the brain, Carla relaxes a little and begins to describe some of her obsessions and compulsions concerning dirt and germs. Nadine also explains the treatment process to Carla and asks her if she would like to give OCD a nasty nickname. Carla decides she will call it "Germy" and agrees to draw a picture of "Germy" over the next week, as she looks out for where, when, and how OCD bothers her.

### GOALS OF SESSION 1

1. Establish rapport.
2. Provide a neurobehavioral framework.
3. Explain the treatment process.
4. Introduce story metaphors.

## ESTABLISH RAPPORT

The patient and one or both parents are present for this session. In describing this first session, we assume that the child has already undergone a careful neuropsychiatric evaluation and has been diagnosed with OCD.

To enlist the child's cooperation in therapy, Session 1 begins with small talk designed to establish rapport. We often ask younger children to choose a game they would like to play at the end of the session. To relieve anxiety, initial questions should focus on the child's background, likes and dislikes, and hobbies rather than on OCD. In this way, the therapist learns what interests and strengths the child brings to treatment.

We state at the outset that the child and family are in a contest or battle with OCD and the goal of treatment is to provide the child with allies and a strategy for "bossing back OCD." We cannot emphasize enough that the tone and content of the entire therapeutic conversation must explicitly and implicitly establish that the therapist is on the side of the child and family against OCD. It is sometimes helpful for therapists to identify what went well or poorly in the treatment of previous patients. We have found that blaming the child or parent, focusing exclusively on drug treatment, or failing to consider comorbid conditions, such as depression, social phobia, or an occult learning disability, characterize most treatment failures. The therapist should also assess the level of understanding that the child and family bring to treatment in order to minimize redundancy, emphasize the main points, and correct faulty assumptions. Once rapport is established, the interview focuses on building a common neurobehavioral framework for understanding OCD.

## PROVIDE A NEUROBEHAVIORAL FRAMEWORK

In the next step, the therapist reviews the current scientific understanding of OCD and places the disorder in a neurobehavioral framework (i.e., "neuro," neurological; "behavioral," manifested in thoughts, feelings, and behaviors). Although we take pains to point out that OCD can be eliminated through actions taken by the child, we also emphasize that OCD is not a bad habit that must be corrected. We help the child and parents understand that OCD is a neurological problem that cannot, in any way, be viewed as the child's "fault" or as something the child could stop "if he or she just tried harder." Instead, we explicitly present OCD as a "short circuit," "brain hiccups," and/or as a "volume control" problem in the brain—whichever metaphor the child finds appealing. Using the child's OCD symptoms as a guide to the discussion, the therapist describes a "worry computer" that inappropriately sends fear cues when no threat is present or turns up the volume on fear cues that do not deserve such attention (see Dialogue 4.1).

The therapist then carefully defines "obsessions" and "compulsions." We explain that obsessions are unwanted thoughts, urges, or images that are accompanied by negative feelings and that compulsions are actions designed to make these thoughts go away and to relieve accompanying negative affects. The therapist illustrates these definitions with examples taken from the child's own OCD symptoms, using other OC symptoms as necessary. In order to focus on the child's strengths, the therapist notes that OCD (described as "brain hiccups") is an illness distinct from the child as a person and does not affect the ability of the rest of the brain (and child) to function normally. Using analogies to other medical illnesses, such as asthma, diabetes, or arthritis, often helps clarify this picture. You would not confuse the symptoms of diabetes with willful misbehavior—there is no reason to do so with OCD either.

Finally, using information from the child's psychiatric or psychological evaluation, including the YBOCS Symptom Checklist, the therapist provides information and answers questions regarding the phenomenology, epidemiology, neurobiology, and appropriate treatment of OCD. For children receiving concurrent pharmacotherapy, the therapist should emphasize the potential synergy of pharmacotherapy and CBT. Jeff Schwartz's description of medications as "water wings" may help set the appropriate tone (Schwartz, 1996) (i.e., just as water wings are helpful when first learning to swim, medications are helpful when implementing CBT and can later be withdrawn when they are no longer needed). Children who learn to view OCD as a "brain hiccup" can more easily let go of the notion that they or their parents are the problem. This formulation is one aspect of linguistically separating OCD from the child (who is thus labeled as an otherwise normal youngster), so that OCD becomes a separate object that can be addressed in treatment. Approaching OCD in this fashion allows the child, family members, and the therapist to become allies against OCD rather than battling with each other over "who is at fault." During this first session, we introduce a set of specific linguistic interventions that will be completed in Session 2, including giving OCD a nickname. Choosing a derogatory epithet for OCD helps make the disorder the problem by setting up a "good guys" versus "bad guys" dichotomy between the child and OCD. Younger children often choose names like "stupid" or "terrible trouble." Somewhat older children may choose a comic book character or a less than favorite adult. Adolescents usually call OCD by its medical name. Once OCD is clearly identified and named as the problem, the treatment process of "bossing back" OCD begins.

*Dialogue 4.1*

NADINE: Carla, there are two aspects of OCD I want to tell you about. The first is that OCD is a problem in the brain. If the brain were a computer, OCD would be one small chip that kept sending out the wrong message, loudly, to the rest of the computer. In other words, one part of the brain sends thoughts, urges, or feelings of fear to you and to the rest of your body when it's not supposed to. Or it might send a *big* fear message instead of a small fear message when something unusual but normal occurs. It is kind of like the brain gets the hiccups, which you experience as OCD. In your case, OCD gives you a *big* fear message concerning normal every-day experiences. For example, when you go into public restrooms, your brain might tell you to be *extra, extra* careful and wash your hands many times, instead of gently reminding you to wash before you leave. These fear messages are called obsessions. The second part of OCD is the action you do to make the fear message go away, such as washing your hands over and over again. These actions are called compulsions, and they actually make OCD stronger because you are doing what OCD wants you to do. Medication can help the first aspect of OCD by turning down the volume a little in that part of your brain. *You* can help with the second part of OCD by bossing OCD back. While we are working together, I will be like your coach and teach you how to boss back OCD.

CARLA: You mean when I wash my hands extra times that hiccups in my brain are telling me to do it?

NADINE: Yes, that's right Carla—particularly since you know it doesn't make any sense, right? It is just like hiccups, and my job is to teach you how to get rid of them. The first thing we'll do is to give OCD a nasty nickname. You can call it anything you would like and if you would like to think it over this week, that's fine too. Do you have any name in mind?

CARLA: I think I'll call it "Germy" because now I know for sure it's silly.

At this point, the therapist may find it helpful to show pictures of brain images before and after treatment and discuss with the child (see Figures 4.1 and 4.2).

## EXPLAIN THE TREATMENT PROCESS

"Bossing back" or "saying no" to OCD is the essence of the treatment process. "Bossing back OCD" requires two things: *allies* and *a battle strategy*, both of which are usually missing when parents and children enter therapy. For the child to be successful in the struggle with OCD, we recruit allies (therapist, parents, teachers, and friends) and provide

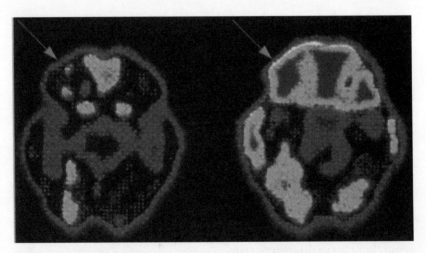

Normal control

Obsessive–compulsive

**FIGURE 4.1.** Positron emission tomography with and without OCD. The arrow points to heightened activity, indicated by more grey in brain areas affected by OCD, such as the orbital–frontal cortex. Used by permission of Jeff Schwartz, UCLA School of Medicine.

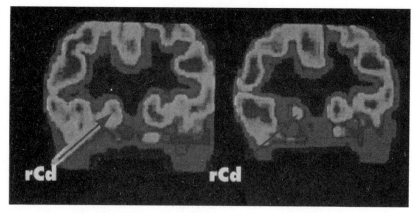

Before CBT                        After CBT

**FIGURE 4.2.** Positron emission tomography in a patient with OCD before and after CBT. The decrease in brain activity (indicated by less grey at the arrow pointing to the right caudate nucleus) parallel the improvement in OCD symptoms with CBT. Used by permission of Jeff Schwartz, UCLA School of Medicine.

clear strategies (CBT techniques). Exposure and response prevention is the core of the "tool kit" the child will use to "boss" OCD; the therapist serves as "coach" to facilitate the process (see Dialogue 4.2).

It is critical for the therapist to be sure the child understands the related concepts of exposure and response prevention in the context of the statement "Who's the boss, you or OCD?" The *exposure* principle states that adequate exposure to a feared stimulus will ultimately reduce anxiety. Exposure requires the child to confront triggers for OCD (e.g., touching a "contaminated" door knob). The *response prevention* principle states that adequate exposure depends on blocking rituals and/or minimizing avoidance behaviors. Technically, response prevention is an extinction procedure (i.e., by removing the negative reinforcing property of the rituals, habituation occurs). In our program, we also define extinction to mean eliminating OCD behaviors by removing parental positive reinforcement. Response prevention takes place when the child refuses to perform the usual anxiety-relieving compulsion (e.g., washing hands or using a tissue to grasp the knob). Extinction occurs when parents ignore the child's compulsive seeking of reassurance or, in this example, refuse to grasp the knob for the child. When explaining exposure and response prevention (E/RP), it is helpful to use examples from the child's own OCD symptoms to clarify the treatment process. The therapist must also make it clear that, although the child will be able to "boss OCD" in the future, he or she is not expected to do so today.

Because E/RP is always threatening for the child, the therapist needs to give two primary assurances: (1) the child will be given a "tool kit" of coping strategies to use when he or she experiences anxiety or other dysphoric affects during E/RP; and (2) treatment will proceed at the child's chosen pace (i.e., the "allies" won't suddenly become enemies by asking the child to do the impossible). When a child is exposed to a feared cue and resists performing the usual compulsive response, he or she will invariably experience increased anxiety and must therefore be prepared to expect, measure, and tolerate that anxiety. The "tool kit," which is introduced in Session 2, provides this preparation. The therapist sets the pace by coaching the child to choose tasks that he or she is ready to face, usually those that the child has already confronted with some success. Using humor links OCD to a different affect and helps alleviate the embarrassment and demoralization children feel as a result of OCD. Since children are frequently secretive about their symptoms, laughing at OCD (not at the child) can help children discuss OCD in a less threatening context and gain trust in the therapist.

While the treatment may proceed slowly, there must always be some movement, however small, toward the goal of giving OCD a less prominent role in the child's life. Otherwise, the therapy itself can come to serve as an avoidance behavior. Thus, therapists must empha-size their intransigence against OCD on the side of the child and stress that this shared attitude will not permit the absence of progress. Stated differently, the therapist should assume that the patient and family are "doing the best they can" at any given point in therapy. This attitude completely avoids the blaming that is inherent in the use of terms such as resistance, denial, or enmeshment, since it assumes that all family members are coping as well as they are able, even if this may not be very skillfully, with OCD. At the same time, the therapist (who controls the structure of the treatment) must insist that the patient and family move toward a more skillful means of bossing back OCD, but at *their* preferred pace, not the therapist's.

During this first session, the therapist gives the child and parents a copy of Handout 1, "Your CBT Program" (provided in Appendix I), and then describes what will happen during each treatment session and briefly illustrates each item in the tool kit (see Dialogue 4.2).

Sharing stories about other children who have successfully completed treatment is often helpful in making the treatment protocol real to the child.

### Dialogue 4.2

NADINE: I will be your coach over the next 4 months and will teach you how to boss back OCD. We will work together each week and you will get to practice what you learn between sessions. You will be able to choose what practice to do. How does that sound so far?

CARLA: That sounds okay.

NADINE: To boss back OCD, we first need to know what OCD looks like and how much of your life is under the control of OCD. Therefore, today and over the next few weeks, we will work together to "map out" OCD. We want to find out what part your life OCD controls, what part you control, and what part is half-and-half. The half-and-half part, where you mostly win but OCD wins some of the time, will be where we start to boss OCD back. Does this mapping idea make sense to you? If you have any questions, please stop me and I'll explain some more. [The therapist may want to show the child the Map Figure (Handout 2, Appendix I) if the child seems to be having difficulty grasping the concept of mapping OCD.]

CARLA: You mean I can make rituals into cities and then try to take them over?

NADINE: That's right, Carla. And while we are mapping OCD, I will give you some tools to help you boss OCD off your map. There are two big tools, and these are the most important. One is called exposure and the second is called response prevention. Before I tell you what these two tools are, I want to assure you that you will be in charge of when and how you use them. We will always boss OCD back at your pace. Now, exposure happens when you do the thing OCD is telling you not to do, like going into a public bathroom and touching the toilet or sink. Response prevention happens when you let yourself feel anxious without doing any compulsions or rituals, like washing your hands over and over again. You may think this will make your fear go up higher and higher, but what actually happens is that gradually your fear and anxiety will go down until they are gone or very, very small. It is a little like riding a roller coaster—the first time you ride one it can feel very scary, but if you keep riding the same roller coaster over and over again, after the third or fourth time, it's not scary any more. [Other examples of how "familiarity breeds contempt" that may be helpful include diving off the high dive, going up a ladder if scared of heights, giving a speech in front of the class, starting middle school, driving a car.] What do you think about this so far?

CARLA: How do I know the anxious feeling will go away? What can I do?

NADINE: I have some other tools to teach you that will help you during the exposure and response prevention. The "fear thermometer" is one tool, which will help you know how high your fear goes and how low it comes down. I will also teach you some relaxation exercises that will help you control your body's fear and tension. Talking back to OCD is another important tool that will help you feel less fear and tension about OCD.

There's one more tool which is very, very important, and that is a sense of humor. OCD likes to be taken very seriously, so the more we can laugh at OCD the better. Remember, as I said before, we will go at your pace, but it is important that we go. It's okay to tackle OCD slowly, little by little, but if you stand still, then OCD wins. That's why I'm here as your coach to encourage you to keep on, so that you can beat OCD. You'd like to do that, right?

CARLA: Yeah, I want to get rid of these silly worries.

## INTRODUCE STORY METAPHORS

The therapist now introduces the idea that the child has a choice about including or excluding OCD from his life story. Past chapters have been taken up with OCD; future chapters need not be. According to Michael White's concept of narrative therapy (White & Epston, 1990), story metaphors are found by selecting out of the totality of the child's experience those aspects (1) that can be readily assembled into an autobiographical or narrative format and (2) that can be used to drive OCD out of the child's life space by discovering unique instances of success in bossing back OCD. When these concepts are presented in this way, children can readily incorporate story metaphors into OCD treatment. Such metaphors stimulate children's hope that they can author a more congenial story—a story without OCD at its center.

## DEVELOPMENTAL CONSIDERATIONS

Developmental considerations (see Chapters 2 and 17 for more detailed discussions) require flexibility on the part of the therapist in adjusting the moment-to-moment conduct of each session to individual differences in each child, although the general format and goals of treatment remain the same for all children. The therapist needs to adjust the level of discourse to the child's or adolescent's level of cognitive functioning, social maturity, and capacity for sustained attention. For example, younger children require more redirection and activities, while older children may be more sensitive to peer issues and will need more opportunity for discussion. Younger children may also appreciate more "play" time as dictated by their attention span and emotional needs. Adolescents often appreciate a more detailed and technical explanation of OCD, while children under 12 or 13 can sometimes be better engaged in the treatment process using story telling or drawing.

## PARENT CHECK-IN

Parents are included in the first session so that the therapist can provide psychoeducation concerning OCD, address their specific concerns, and provide support. This session also gives the therapist the opportunity to assess the degree to which OCD involves each parent in the child's rituals or avoidance strategies, the associated level of negative affect, and the coping strategies the family members are using to deal with OCD.

Since a successful outcome of treatment depends on the cooperation of parents, it is especially important to address any questions that parents might have regarding OCD or its treatment. It is also important at the start of treatment for the therapist, as the expert in the treatment of OCD, to encourage parents to surrender control for managing the child's OCD to the therapist, so that control can then be successfully transferred back to the child and parents as they learn to deal skillfully with OCD as the therapy proceeds.

The following points deserve emphasis:

• Parents should be encouraged to align with child and therapist against OCD. In this way, they form a team who can work together to develop a "battle plan" for fighting OCD. It is useful to emphasize with parents that CBT and E/RP are not a "just do it" approach, but are used gradually at the child's own pace. Parents are also informed that their role in helping their youngster resist OCD will increase and become more specific as treatment proceeds.

• At this session, parents frequently request specific guidance regarding how they can best respond to OCD. Parents should be given copies of the "Tips for Parents" booklet and the "Guide for Patients and Families" from the *Expert Consensus Treatment Guidelines for Obsessive–Compulsive Disorder* (March, Frances, et al., 1997) (copies of which are provided in Appendix III) and asked to read them. The therapist can also suggest that they may want to read other books on the resource list (Appendix III) and to consult with advocacy groups, such as the OC Foundation. It is also helpful to point out that patience is a cardinal virtue, especially at the beginning of treatment.

• The therapist should explain to parents that punishment makes OCD worse and harder to resist and that OCD is *not* bad behavior, but rather an illness. Everyone in the family should try to respond to each other as much as possible in a spirit of generosity and kindness.

• Parents should be told that their feedback is encouraged throughout treatment and that the therapist will check in with them at the beginning and end of each session.

During Session 1, parents are instructed (1) to stop giving advice about OCD and (2) to pay attention to elements of their child's behavior that are not affected by OCD. This requires that parents respond with patience and kindness, cooperating with rituals where necessary, while at the same time switching the focus of attention from OCD to the child's strengths.

## EVALUATION

Before moving on to homework, the therapist may wish to spend a few minutes on the NIMH Global OC Scale and the Clinical Global Impairment Scale. During the second week, the Clinical Global Improvement Scale will also be included.

## HOMEWORK

General Principles

Just as tennis or ballet lessons require practice, a child with OCD must practice "bossing back" OCD both during sessions in the therapist's office and in homework assignments. The therapist must carefully explain these homework assignments to the child and emphasize the importance of bossing OCD each day, while also providing reassurance that the child and therapist will decide on homework tasks together. The therapist should inform the child that the homework is time limited and specific and will be under the child's control. The therapist should make sure that the child understands that he or she will choose only those E/RP tasks that he or she feels quite ready to perform. As explained in Sessions 2 and 3, the "map" of OCD is the primary source for selecting homework tasks, so it is important to work hard to generate an accurate map of OCD.

Homework Assignments

Unlike homework assignments for most sessions, this session's assignment is prescriptive.

• To actively reinforce the concept of making OCD the identified problem, the therapist asks the child to choose a funny nickname for OCD (if he or she has not already done so) that the patient and therapist will use to refer to OCD during the remainder of the treatment. Children (especially adolescents) who prefer to use the term OCD rather than a nickname should, of course, be allowed to do so.

• Anticipating Session 2, the therapist also asks the child to notice where OCD wins and where he or she wins so that they can start to make a map of OCD at the next visit.

• The child and parents should be asked to review the materials given to them during this first session: the "Outline of Treatment," "Tips for Parents" booklet, and the "Guide for Patients and Families" from the OCD Expert Consensus Guidelines (copies of which are provided in Appendices I and III). The therapist should also suggest that they may wish to peruse other books on the resource list (Appendix III) and to consult with advocacy groups, such as the OC Foundation.

• Parents should be instructed to stop giving advice about the unreasonableness of OCD. Instead, since OCD symptoms will take some time to remit with treatment, it is best in the meantime if parents simply respond to their child's OCD symptoms with patience, generosity, and kindness.

• To minimize negative interactions, which form a barrier to effective CBT, parents should also be instructed to redirect their attention away from OCD to those things that go well for their child (i.e., differential reinforcement of other behavior [DRO]).

• If needed, parents may be coached on how to work with teachers to encourage them to assume the same compassionate framework for approaching OCD.

Chapter 5

# Session 2: Introducing the "Tool Kit"

When Carla returns for her second CBT session, she tells Nadine that she has tried to resist Germy a few times during the past week, telling it to go away. She did so once when someone brushed up against her at school, telling herself, "I'm not going to wash my hands—that's just my brain hiccuping." Carla reports that she felt a little anxious at first, but that the feeling of worry then went away, and she was especially glad to be able to stay with her friends. Carla brings in her picture of Germy to show Nadine, but wants to take it home with her again to hang it on the bathroom door so she can remember to "boss it back." Carla tells Nadine that during the past week she has tried to notice all the places and ways Germy bothers her, so that she is ready to begin to "map out" her obsessions and compulsions.

## GOALS OF SESSION 2

1. Make OCD the problem.
2. Begin mapping OCD.
3. Introduce the fear thermometer (includes introducing the concepts of talking back to OCD and E/RP).

## REVIEW HOMEWORK

The therapist should ask the child to describe the nickname he or she has chosen for OCD (if one was not already decided on during the first session) and to explain why it was picked. It is especially important to be sure that the chosen nickname helps the child feel optimistic and in control of OCD. Ask about the history associated with the nickname and ask the child how he or she has used it in conversations about OCD (both internal and with others) since the last visit. As mentioned earlier, watch out for nicknames that demonize OCD (i.e., make OCD large, dangerous, and powerful) or that exacerbate symptoms. For example, it is best to stay away from nicknames such as "slash" or "torture man" unless it is clear that their derivation is lighthearted. Some nicknames, such as "sicko," although funny and ultimately helpful, may also trigger OCD symptoms. For example, a child with germ worries may experience the thought of "sicko" as a trigger for OCD symptoms. While this isn't necessarily a bad thing, it is important to ask the child if using the nickname made OCD mad and, if so, if he or she was successful in resisting the urge to ritualize. Finally, be sure that your use of the nickname does not have a different effect than your patient's use of it (e.g., making the child feel mocked or provoking symptoms).

## MAKE OCD THE PROBLEM

Using the child's name for OCD, the therapist should then ask a set of very general questions about how OCD has been bossing the child around and how the child has successfully bossed OCD back. Questions the therapist might ask include:

- How has OCD bossed you around this week?
- How does OCD mess things up for you at home? At school? With your friends?
- How have you said "No" to OCD?
- Can you give me an example of how you beat up on OCD this week?
- When you "beat up" OCD, how did it feel? What did you say to yourself?
- Who helps you boss OCD back?

- How would *[name a hero likely to appeal to the child]* boss OCD around?
- Who do you most want to know about your success in writing OCD out of your story?
- What will your life without OCD look like?

Framing questions in this fashion reinforces the idea that OCD is external to the child so that the child is no longer seen as the problem. Equally important, this approach identifies and builds on the child's strengths and so encourages him or her to resist OCD. To gather the maximum amount of information and avoid embarrassing the child, questioning should proceed from the general to the specific.

## BEGIN MAPPING OCD

During Session 2, we develop the idea of a road map to OCD and introduce the concept of a transition zone between territory controlled by OCD and territory under the child's control. During Sessions 3 and 4, we will complete the process of mapping OCD, including the specific obsessions and compulsions, triggers, and avoidance behaviors that comprise the stimulus hierarchy (see below). We use the YBOCS Symptom Checklist and patient's history to inventory the child's OCD symptoms and the fear thermometer to generate subjective units of discomfort scores (SUDS) for each item on a stimulus hierarchy. The child will then learn to rank his or her OCD symptoms from the easiest to hardest to "boss back," thus generating the stimulus hierarchy. After the child's OCD symptoms are ranked on the stimulus hierarchy, it is straightforward to understand where the child's life territory is free from OCD, where OCD and the child each "win" some of the time, and where the child cedes control to OCD. In this process, we are chiefly concerned with identifying the region where the child is *sometimes* able to successfully "boss back" OCD, which we term the *transition* or *work zone*. It is a transition zone in that it defines the place where OCD and the child both win some of the time; it is a work zone in that this is the region that will serve as a source for choosing E/RP targets for the child to become 100% successful in resisting OCD. You and the child may call it either the transition or work zone, but it is important to communicate both concepts at this point in the session. In practice, the transition/work zone is usually defined by the lower end of the stimulus hierarchy. As treatment proceeds, the transition zone provides a dependable guide for the child to use when selecting targets for graded E/RP.

The therapist should describe for the child the two basic "flavors" of OCD, one involving negative affects (for example, fear of harm, disgust, or guilt) and the other involving a felt need for having things "just so" (for example, symmetry urges and feelings of incompleteness) (see Dialogue 5.1). The first category can be easily understood by analogy to normal feelings. It is the context (inappropriate to the circumstances), timing (inappropriate to age), and impairment (the obsessions/feelings serve no useful purpose) that distinguish OCD from normal obsessive–compulsive thoughts, feelings, and behaviors. "Just so" feelings can be made comprehensible in the same way (e.g., using the analogy of scratching a mosquito bite, except the itch never seems to end). Compulsions are actions designed to alleviate these internal dysphorias, anxiety, and "just so" feelings and needs. Patients may have both types of symptoms. Be sure to use examples from the child's own OCD symptoms and to draw on examples from your own treatment experience to illustrate the nature of OCD.


## Dialogue 5.1

NADINE: OCD usually comes in two different "flavors." Just like flavors of ice cream taste different, flavors of OCD feel different. One flavor of OCD bosses kids (and adults) around by making them feel afraid of harm or making them afraid something very bad will happen. The other OCD flavor bosses by making people feel they need to do things "just so" or get things "just right." What flavor is Germy, do you think?

CARLA: Oh, I know mine is the first flavor—I'm afraid of something bad happening.


After the specific feelings driving OCD in the child are understood, the therapist can begin mapping OCD's present influence, with emphasis on identifying the transition zone. When explaining these concepts, be sure to use examples from the child's symptoms to make the point that OCD proceeds from trigger to thought or feeling to ritual (e.g., when Carla sees a doorknob, this provokes thoughts about Germy, which in turn lead to the urge to wash). In addition to using the child's own experiences to illustrate these concepts, the therapist can also draw on the experiences of other children with OCD and explain how other children with similar OCD symptoms were able to push OCD out of the picture using the techniques they learned in treatment. It also never hurts to remind the child that you will teach her specific techniques to help combat OCD.

The therapist should then introduce the map metaphor shown in Handout 2 (Appendix I). This map differentiates territory controlled by and free from OCD and illustrates how the child can shrink the territory controlled by OCD by picking E/RP targets from the part of the map called the *transition* or *work zone* (see Dialogue 5.2). The territory occupied by OCD can be described as a place no one would ever want to visit, the child's territory as a vacation paradise. To identify territory controlled by OCD, it is helpful to use information from the YBOCS Symptom Checklist that was obtained during the child's initial evaluation. The transition zone is the territory where the child is already successfully resisting OCD some of the time (i.e., where resistance occurs with at least "some control" as specified on items 4 and 5 of the YBOCS). The transition/work zone will serve at the primary guide for selecting E/RP targets. In this way, we use the map metaphor to introduce the concept of a *stimulus hierarchy*—a listing of OC symptoms ranked according to difficulty for exposure and response prevention—and to project into the future how the child will move up the hierarchy from easy to more difficult elements. In addition, the map metaphor shows the child how the therapist intends to be his or her ally against OCD, with both occupying territory free of OCD.

## Dialogue 5.2

NADINE: Kids with OCD mostly try to make those fears, feelings, and urges go away by doing a ritual or by avoiding OCD's territory. To know how to beat up on OCD, we need to identify OCD's territory and what rituals or habits help out OCD. This week and next week we are going to draw a map of Germy. There are three parts to this map. The first part is where Germy always wins and has control (*draws a large circle to indicate OCD's territory*). The second part is where you always win, or where Germy almost never tries to boss you around (*draws a smaller circle next to the large one*). The third part is in the middle and you and I can call it the transition or work zone. This is where sometimes Germy wins and sometimes you win (*draws an arrow between the two circles*). [The therapist may want to use other analogies to further explain the transition zone, such as the image of playing tug-of-war.] Can you tell me about a time when Germy tried to boss you around, but you did not do the usual ritual or habit—in other words, a time when you bossed back Germy? We call this region on the map the transition or work zone because it is the place where you and OCD both win some of the time and because it is in this region where you will choose E/RP targets to resist OCD. Some kids call it the TZ for short. What would you like to call it?

CARLA: I think I'll call it the T-zone.

## INTRODUCE THE FEAR THERMOMETER

After introducing the concept of mapping OCD, we next present a tool for rating the anxiety associated with specific OCD symptoms. It is important for the child to be able to distinguish between levels of anxiety when participating in E/RP tasks, since the child must tolerate elevated levels of discomfort and stay with the experience until the discomfort level decreases significantly. The extent to which a person becomes frightened or upset is usually rated in terms of a SUDS score. We use a "fear thermometer" to establish the functional equivalent of the SUDS score (see Handout 3 in Appendix I). The fear thermometer provides the child with a tool for measuring (or rating) anxiety or other dysphoric affects. The fear thermometer is also used during exposure tasks to measure the child's anxiety until it attenuates, which in turn documents the success of the treatment strategy. Used as a numerical scale, the fear thermometer also helps the child rank specific OCD symptoms according to their potency or difficulty when presented as targets for E/RP. The fear thermometer helps the child be more realistic about his or her probable responses to OCD triggers (i.e., all fear isn't absolute terror and all anger isn't necessarily rage). Since OCD fears decrease with treatment, fear thermometer ratings for items remaining on the stimulus hierarchy may need to be updated during any given session.

During this second session, the child, with the therapists' help, makes a first attempt at ranking currently identified symptoms in hierarchical order of difficulty using the fear thermometer rating to judge the anxiety associated with resisting each potential OCD trigger. During Session 3, the therapist will address mapping OCD in greater detail. The purpose during Session 2 is simply to introduce the idea of rating items on a stimulus hierarchy, which will be completed during the next session using the fear thermometer.

Show the child a picture of a thermometer labeled "Fear" (Handout 3, Appendix I). Explain that fears can be stronger or weaker and that we're going to use this thermometer to show how to describe different levels of fears. Put numbers from 1 to 10 on the thermometer. (Instead of numbers, very young children may prefer to color the thermometer up to his or her anxiety level, thus using it as a visual analog scale.) Although one can begin with OCD triggers, it is usually better to start by considering other triggers for anxiety. Tell the child that level 10 represents the most afraid he or she has ever been (i.e., absolutely terrified or too scared to move). Give an example of a 10 experience from your experience working with other children or from your own life. Point out that number 1 on the fear thermometer is the least afraid and most secure the child has ever felt (i.e., relaxed, asleep, "chilled out"). Find an example for this anchor point as well. Go through the same process for a "5" on the fear thermometer. If you can find examples easily, fill in the intermediate points as well. If the child has difficulty precisely locating the fears on the scale (e.g., because of the indecisiveness that may be associated with OCD), the therapist should ask for a "best guess" or a general rating of low, medium, or high.

After teaching the idea that fears can be ranked, the therapist should give the child a new blank thermometer. Make a list of five to eight OCD symptoms as well as their triggers and the obsessions and rituals associated with them and rank these from the most easily resisted to the most difficult to resist using the fear thermometer to establish the ranking. Use the Symptom Hierarchy List (see Handout 4 in Appendix I) to list these symptoms. Ask the child about how much he or she resists each OCD trigger/symptom, and when resisted, how much control he or she has over OCD. Use this information to locate a trigger or two (very low on the hierarchy) that the child resists successfully more than half the time. Point out that this is where the transition or work zone is located and comment that it is easy to beat OCD here, but much harder high up on the hierarchy, which is why you'll start in the transition zone. Ask what it would take to win against OCD 100% of the time for those items in the transition zone. While it may be tempting to structure an E/RP task at this point, resist the temptation, since it may prove to be poorly targeted. Let the child know that the two of you will use a refined version of the hierarchy to set up the first E/RP task at the next session (see Dialogue 5.3).

The fear thermometer, which is used to place symptoms on the symptom hierarchy; should be kept current and new symptoms added and old symptoms reevaluated as needed. (Note that by plotting fear thermometer ratings for each exposure target across sessions, the therapist ends up generating a single-subject multiple baseline design in which each OCD symptom is a single baseline assessed with the fear thermometer).

## Dialogue 5.3

NADINE: Carla, let's look at the fear thermometer together.

CARLA: That's funny (*laughs*).

NADINE: Can you think of something really scary—not about OCD, but something else—that would be a 10 on the fear thermometer?

CARLA: Yes, getting left alone at the State Fair. That would definitely be a 10.

NADINE: How about something that would be a 1 or a 0?

CARLA: Maybe, watching TV, like Barney, yuk!

NADINE: Okay, how about something in the middle, where if you forced yourself to do it, you'd get pretty scared, but not nearly so bad as a 10?

CARLA: Oh, that's easy. I went on the roller coaster at the State Fair, but only after everyone else went on it a bunch of times. [Nadine uses this example to draw a parallel with planned exposure and minimizing avoidance with OCD, and how this will lead to habituation of OCD fears. Carla and Nadine then fill in the middle sections—6–9 and 2–4.]

NADINE: Okay, Carla, now that you get the idea of how fears and worries can be ranked from 1 to 10 in terms of how scared you'd get, let's do the same thing for OCD.

CARLA: Okay.

NADINE: Can you think of an OCD trigger, say, something like [uses an example from Carla's symptoms] that would be at the top of the list, say a 9 or a 10?

CARLA: Yep, how about touching my aunt who has cancer.

NADINE: How about at the very bottom, where you are almost always able to do the opposite of what OCD tells you to do? [Carla and Nadine proceed to fill in some more OCD symptoms on the hierarchy, including the main classes of OCD symptoms that bother Carla. No attempt should be made to complete the hierarchy at this point, since the idea today is simply to get the idea across.]

NADINE: That's terrific, Carla.

CARLA: I'm glad you know what's too hard for me to do now, but I wish my Mom understood better.

NADINE: We'll use the fear thermometer to show her, okay?

## DEVELOPMENTAL CONSIDERATIONS

In sharpening the distinction between the child and OCD, humor on the part of the therapist is essential in helping the child see how silly and bossy OCD really is. Gentle humor on the part of the child also helps by linking a different affect to the OCD symptoms, thereby rendering OCD less powerful in the mind of the child. Likewise, the therapist's use of humorous metaphoric language, such as using the OCD nickname, models for the child the reality of OCD as a manageable problem separate from the child. The therapist should, however, keep two caveats in mind when externalizing and poking fun at OCD. First, the aim of giving OCD a nickname is to bring it down to size and to make it the object of treatment. If, however, the child chooses a nickname that demonizes OCD (i.e., ends up making it bigger and stronger), then the therapist will have failed to achieve the goal. Second, externalizing OCD and poking fun at the disorder is a weak exposure task in which the child is explicitly signaling his or her willingness to resist OCD. In some children, even this degree of exposure is threatening and so must be carefully rationed.

## PARENT CHECK-IN

It is not desirable at this point for a parent to become involved in the exposure tasks or to assist with response prevention. Most children with OCD have received unhelpful advice from parents. Parents may also have become involved in the child's OCD rituals. During later sessions, the child will be given the freedom to decide when he or she is ready for a coach at home and to choose who will perform that role. As stated previously, parents should be supported and their feedback encouraged, but their primary role at this time is that of a cheerleader. It can be helpful for some parents to address their own feelings of anxiety in the presence of OCD. Parents should also be encouraged to praise the child for resisting OCD, while at the same time refocusing their attention on positive elements in the child's life (DRO). If necessary, use the child's fear thermometer to illustrate the fact that many OCD symptoms will not be approached via E/RP until much later in treatment. For these symptoms, reinforce the idea that the child will resist as best he or she can, in order not to inconvenience family members, and that parents should be patient and sympathetic in response. Let parents know that Sessions 7 and 12 will be devoted to disentangling family members from OCD.

## EVALUATION

Near the end of the session, spend a few minutes obtaining ratings on the NIMH Global OC Scale and on the CGI scales.

## HOMEWORK

The homework given at Session 2 is again prescriptive:

- The child is encouraged to act as a sleuth to detect OCD triggers and to list and rate them using the fear thermometer and the Symptom List, which are given to the child to take home. Adolescents may also be given the YBOCS Symptom Checklist to use as a guide. In this way, the child reinforces making OCD the problem, as well as continues the process of mapping the state of OCD at the present time.
- Parents are encouraged to continue being supportive and to practice DRO.

# Chapter 6

## Session 3: Mapping OCD

This week Carla returns carrying a little notebook in which she has been writing down the places Germy bothers her. Using the Symptom List, she has ranked several triggers that result in an urge to wash her hands. These include school books, public restrooms, household cleansers, people who are sick, and doorknobs. During the session, Nadine and Carla refine the Symptom List and give each trigger an anxiety rating using the fear thermometer. Nadine also helps Carla identify what kind of thoughts and feelings she is having before and during the compulsion. Carla learns some new ways of thinking this week. She also decides to reward herself with an ice cream cone each time she practices "bossing back" Germy.

### GOALS OF SESSION 3

1. Begin cognitive training.
2. Continue mapping OCD and review the symptom list.
3. Learn to use rewards as a strategy.

### REVIEW HOMEWORK

This session begins with a review of the symptom list the child has begun to identify. If the child was unable to write down symptoms since the previous session, spend time at the beginning of this session doing the homework together. Parents may also participate in this process at the beginning of the session. Reinforce the child's compliance both in completing the homework and in participating during the session. Tell the child that you'll return to the Symptom List toward the end of the session, but that first you want to teach some tools for talking back to OCD.

## BEGIN COGNITIVE TRAINING

While E/RP by itself is sufficient to decrease OCD symptoms, many children lack the cognitive framework to succeed at E/RP even though they know what to do. When actually undertaking an E/RP task, children and adolescents (perhaps more than adults) tend to engage in negative self-talk that disables them and empowers OCD. Thus, it turns out to be very helpful to provide the child with a cognitive strategy for "bossing back" OCD. Targets for CT include reinforcing accurate information regarding OCD and its treatment, cognitive resistance, and self-administered positive reinforcement and encouragement. We use three techniques, each well validated in the CBT literature, to meet these goals: (1) constructive self-talk, (2) cognitive restructuring, and (3) cultivating detachment. Each technique must be individualized to match the child's specific OCD symptoms and must mesh with the child's cognitive abilities, developmental stage, and individual preference among the three techniques. It is generally best to develop a tailored "short form" of cognitive techniques that the child can use on a regular basis during E/RP.

### Constructive Self-Talk

By now the therapist should have a general idea regarding the child's customary pattern of self-talk in the face of OCD. Some children are eternal optimists and go down swinging after tackling E/RP targets that are clearly too difficult; more often, children with OCD are unrealistically pessimistic, attributing all power to OCD and little to themselves. Despite seeing themselves as powerless in the face of OCD, most children are very critical of themselves for engaging in rituals, especially when doing so causes failure in school or problems at home. Such punitive self-talk contributes to the overall anxiety experienced before, during, and after exposure tasks and reduces the chance that E/RP will be successful. Negative self-statements are especially common in children who have internalizing temperaments or comorbid anxiety and depressive disorders. (When these associated conditions are present, a combination of pharmacotherapy and CBT is more often necessary to reverse the child's habitual pattern of negative cognitions.).

Identifying and correcting unhelpful self-talk is crucial in increasing motivation for E/RP. The general approach relies on replacing maladaptive cognitions, whether overly optimistic or pessimistic, with realistic self-statements that emphasize the child's ability to cope with OCD using the tools being taught in treatment. Take, for example, a youngster with contamination fears and washing rituals who chooses to decrease her usual 2-hour shower by 15 minutes as a homework task. If her internal self-statements prior to the exposure task are "I won't be able to do this. What if I take an even longer shower?", then the likelihood of her actually attempting the exposure task decreases significantly. To decrease the child's general anxiety and increase motivation to practice the exposure task, she might instead consciously think "This task will be difficult, but I can handle this much anxiety this one time. I'll use my tool kit."

Another form of constructive self-talk, which is made possible by the effort to externalize OCD, involves the child's conversation with OCD itself, which we call "talking back to OCD." Here the child simply refuses to give in to OCD, talking back to it in a positive, forceful fashion. This reinforces the idea that OCD is external to the child (preserving insight) and increases the motivation to comply with E/RP. Bossing back OCD in conversation can be difficult, especially when the child directly challenges the obsessions with statements such as "I won't get sick if I touch this faucet," that themselves have the potential to elicit OCD symptoms. Under these circumstances, it is sometimes helpful to suggest that the child use more general "talking back " strategies, such as, "Go jump in a lake OCD, I'm the boss" or "Can't catch me this time, OCD."

In both instances, the overall idea is for the child to realistically assess the difficulty of resisting OCD, for example, saying, "This will be hard, but I can do it—I've done it before," rather than asserting that an E/RP task is either impossible or fabulously easy.

## Cognitive Restructuring

OCD symptoms that are driven by negative affects—such as fear, guilt, or disgust—benefit from formal cognitive restructuring. The first part of the process involves analyzing the child's catastrophic estimations of danger. The second part involves looking at the child's perceived responsibility for the occurrence of the catastrophe. In both steps, the faulty assumptions underlying the child's obsessions are directly confronted, first by the therapist in conversation with the child, and later by the child during E/RP tasks.

Overestimation of risk may result from an overestimation of the probability that an event will occur, of the cost of the resulting consequences, or of personal responsibility for the dread outcome. For example, a child might have a hateful thought, which provokes the obsession that he and his family will go to hell, which in turn causes the child to engage in praying r'_uals to relieve the obsession and accompanying anxiety. In this example, the child behaves as though the trigger (the hateful thought) has a 100% chance of causing an adverse consequence (hell), which will be catastrophic, and that he alone is responsible for the dread outcome. In general, the probabilistic argument regarding risk likelihood is difficult to understand, especially for younger children. The therapist should therefore dispense with such probabilistic arguments and instead focus on addressing overresponsibility unless risk estimation is clearly applicable and helpful for the particular child.

Cognitively restructuring such thoughts is a remarkably straightforward process that depends on moving back and forth between what "OCD says" and what the child actually estimates as a reasonable probability of danger. The goal is for the child to identify the faulty assumptions elicited by OCD so that he or she can then disregard them. The obsession is mapped out according to the probable sequence of events that the child thinks will lead to the catastrophic outcome. Next, the therapist asks the child to estimate the overall chances of the catastrophe happening (e.g., 1 in 10, 1 in 100, 1 in 1000). These probabilities are then compared with the original estimate, generating a convincing "proof" that the risk estimate provided by OCD doesn't make sense.

Even with very small risks, some children and adolescents feel as though they are still responsible for keeping a dreaded outcome from happening (i.e., if it happens it is their fault). To address the issue of overresponsibility, the therapist uses a pie chart (see example in Figure 6.1) to brainstorm with the child concerning what factors may contribute to the occurrence of the feared catastrophe. Once each potential cause has been listed, the adolescent is asked to determine the percentage of responsibility each factor holds vis-à-vis the dreaded outcome. The youngster then determines the amount that is rightfully his or her responsibility. An adolescent who originally thought he was 100% responsible for causing his father's car accident finds that he is

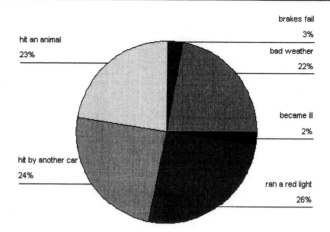

**FIGURE 6.1.** Reasons why Dad had a car accident.

only 1% responsible, if that. In this way, the earlier "proof" regarding risk is extended to demonstrate that the attribution of responsibility elicited by OCD is massively inflated. Armed with such "proof," the adolescent may now be more willing to try an exposure task to verify the prediction that indeed nothing bad will happen if he or she does the opposite of what OCD requires.

Dialogue 6.1 illustrates how Nadine walks Carla through cognitively restructuring her fear of germy plants. Before doing this exercise, Carla was convinced that touching a plant might cause her mother's death.

### Dialogue 6.1

NADINE: Carla, what is the chance that your mother will get sick if you touch her after touching a plant?

CARLA: Germy tells me that it is 100%, but I know that it is not very likely that she'll get sick. After all, she hasn't been sick for several years.

NADINE: If she becomes sick, what is the chance that it will be a fatal illness?

CARLA: Well, Germy says she'll die for sure, but it will probably just be a head cold.

NADINE: Let's say that she becomes deathly ill—I hope it won't happen, but, on rare occasions, people your mother's age do get very sick, don't they? How likely is it that she became ill because you touched a plant and then touched your mother?

CARLA: Zero. I know I wouldn't be responsible. It is just that Germy tries to make me feel that way.

NADINE: What might you say if Germy tries to pull this one over on you again?

CARLA: It isn't very likely that Mom will get sick, and if she does, it won't be bad anyway, and it certainly won't be my fault, so sorry Germy, I just won't buy it.


## Cultivating Nonattachment

Confronting OCD through "talking back" or cognitive restructuring involves taking OCD on its terms. An alternative strategy, popularized by Jeff Schwartz in his book *Brain Lock* (1996), relies on cultivating nonattachment from OCD. Cultivating nonattachment meshes very nicely with narrative approaches to externalizing the problem, such as giving OCD a nasty nickname, and is especially helpful for patients who tend to lose their bearings when they are anxious. Based on work by Paul Salkovskis and colleagues, it also appears that attempts to suppress or neutralize aversive thoughts may make them worse (Salkovskis, Westbrook, Davis, Jeavons, & Gledhill, 1997). Try not to think of an elephant; you'll soon get the idea. In turn, cultivating nonattachment or rational nonsuppression may help to dispel OCD thoughts by facilitating the individual's ability to disengage attention from the emotionally aversive cognitive intrusions that characterize an attack of OCD.

The basic idea is simple: OCD is just a brain hiccup (or, looked at another way, an automatic thought habit) that comes and goes in its own time, so we simply ask patients to see OCD as though it is "just a cloud in the sky," "a fish swimming by in an aquarium," or "a bunch of crazy monkeys up in a tree." In each case, OCD, clouds, goldfish, or goofy monkeys inexorably appear and pass away without any intervention being necessary except noting that the phenomenon in question is again present for a limited time. Stated differently, struggling against OCD sometimes seems to make OCD symptoms worse, so why not just let it come and go without reacting? Eventually, OCD simply disappears with this strategy, since the conditions that produce OCD (avoidance, high levels of affect, and rituals) no longer prevail.

Working with OCD in this fashion involves teaching the child four simple self-statements to use when OCD makes an appearance. First, the child says something like "It's just OCD again," recognizing the obsessions as OCD and not as meaningful self-statements. Sometimes, generating a friendly "Hi [whatever nickname the child has chosen for OCD]" helps reduce the tendency to react emotionally to the OCD symptom. Second, the child makes the statement "My brain is hiccuping again," explicitly recognizing that what we call OCD arises because of misfiring circuits in the central nervous system. Third, the child says "These hiccups are not in themselves important," implying that no response other than patient endurance is necessary because the content of OCD is meaningless. Finally, given meaningless symptoms that will pass away on their own if nothing is done, the child says "I guess I'll go do something pleasant while OCD goes away." Note that these steps imply no need either to avoid OCD triggers or to undertake rituals (i.e., they include E/RP by definition), so it is not surprising that following this program leads to symptom habituation. When working with OCD symptoms in this way, it is helpful to put the four steps down on a card in the child's own words so that he or she can use them whenever OCD symptoms arise.

### Short-Form Cognitive Training

Most children end up merging parts of all three cognitive techniques—constructive self-talk, cognitive restructuring, and cultivating detachment. Having determined which techniques are most acceptable to (and useful for) a particular child, we usually provide a specific step-by-step strategy for thinking about OCD when doing an exposure task. For some children, listing the steps on a 3" × 5" card that can be used during E/RP is helpful. Carla, for example, might notice that she has been worrying about whether or not she can touch a certain doorknob. Step one would be to tell herself that this worry is simply OCD (or Germy), thus distinguishing between the obsession (her mother will get sick) and the compulsion (avoiding her mother and washing). Step two would be to remind herself that she doesn't have to pay any attention to Germy since it is just her brain playing tricks on her. Step three involves reminding herself that the discomfort she experiences when touching the doorknob will go away in a little while so she doesn't need to do the ritual. Step four is to choose to focus her thoughts and/or actions on something besides OCD, such as the soccer game she will play that afternoon, while she waits for the OCD symptoms to abate.

Talking back to OCD is important not only for the child but also for parents, family members, and friends who are also being "bossed around" by OCD. These strategies can be taught to family members who may be tempted to respond to the child's symptoms with unskillful coping strategies.

## CONTINUE MAPPING OCD AND REVIEW THE SYMPTOM LIST

During Session 3, we finish mapping OCD's influence in the child's life both loosely across narrative time (i.e., in past, present, and future) and, most important, in greater detail related to the child's current experience. In this way, we finish filling in the Symptom List (stimulus hierarchy) begun in Session 2. Since OCD symptoms that are untreated or inadequately treated may worsen and cause needless anguish for the child and chagrin for the therapist, careful identification of all OCD symptoms and related behaviors is an essential prerequisite to adequate treatment.

Mapping OCD begins with identifying past and present obsessions and compulsions using the YBOCS Symptom Checklist as a starting point. Current obsessions and corresponding compulsions are then mapped along with their specific triggers, associated avoidance behaviors, time taken, distress, interference with different functional domains (e.g., with peers, at school, or at home), motivation and ability to resist, and finally, incorporation of other people into rituals. Each symptom complex consisting of trigger, obsession, and corresponding compulsion is then ranked on the stimulus hierarchy according to its fear thermometer score and the child's perception of the difficulty of resisting or "bossing back" OCD. An example of a Symptom List (stimulus hierarchy) is shown in Table 6.1. For some patients with complex symptom arrays spanning diverse subtypes of OCD, this process may be better served by using separate hierarchy lists. For example, a patient with contamination fears and washing rituals, fears of sinning and praying rituals, and symmetry/exactness urges and arranging/repeating rituals may do best with one master hierarchy and three separate hierarchies for specific classes of symptoms that each provide sufficient detail to accurately define the transition/work zone.

During this part of the session, the therapist encourages the child to describe all the details of his or her OCD, especially those external triggers that signal OCD's territory. The therapist should pay special attention to objects, people, and places that are avoided as these too represent triggers for OCD. In this way, the therapist and child together

**TABLE 6.1.** Sample Symptom Hierarchy

| Trigger | Obsession | Compulsion | Fear temperature |
|---|---|---|---|
| Touching the bathroom sink | "I'll get germs on my hands and something bad will happen to anyone I touch." | Wash hands five times or avoid touching the sink | 9–10 |
| Touching the toilet | (same) | Avoids touching and washes five times after using the bathroom | 9–10 |
| Using a friend's bathroom | "I'll get their family's germs will give them to my family who will get sick and die." | Avoid going over to the friend's house for any length of time when you may have to use the bathroom | 8 |
| Touching a plant then eating something | "There may be chemicals and I may get sick and die." | Wash five times before eating | 7 |
| Touching my mouth with my fingers | "I'll get sick and die from the germs on my hands." | Wash hands every time fingers touch mouth | 6 |
| Touching doorknobs | "My hands will get other people's germs and then something bad will happen." | Use shirt, coat or tissue to cover handle when opening door | 6 |
| Eating a cookie with bare hands | "I'll get sick and maybe die if my hand touches the cookie and I eat it." | Hold cookie with the wrapper while eating | 5 |
| Touching handles on the sink | "I'll get germs on my hands again and then I will have to wash again so that nothing bad will happen." | Use paper towel to turn handles on and off; rewash if touch by accident | 4–5 |

**TABLE 6.1** (*cont.*)

| Trigger | Obsession | Compulsion | Fear temperature |
|---|---|---|---|
| Petting the dog | "The dog's germs will spread everywhere and someone will get sick and die." | Only pet the dog with gloves on, or wash five times after petting | 3 |
| Touching a plant | "There may be some chemicals on the plant that will cause someone I touch to get sick." | Avoid plant or wash hands after touching | 2 |

begin to generate a picture of the "topography" of OCD (i.e., what OCD looks like and how much territory in the child's life OCD controls). The therapist should also pay special attention to life domains that are not violated by OCD, since it is here that the therapist can identify and build on the child's strengths. Especially important are situations the child enjoys or those in which he or she at least takes risks. Note that risk taking can then be made a part of E/RP.

It helps if the therapist poses questions in a way that alleviates embarrassment. Very specific, matter-of-fact questions that address both the symptom and the child's experience of the symptom are especially useful. For example, the therapist might ask:

- Tell me more about "silly worries" you have.
- Do you find that you have to wash your hands over and over again, even though it makes no sense?
- When you wash your hands, do you have do it in a certain way each time? How?
- Do you count when you wash?
- Other children with this OCD symptom sometimes shower a lot or have to wash in a certain way. How about you?
- Since OCD forced its way in here, how did you manage to keep it out of (name another area)?

By asking very specific questions, the therapist permits the child to volunteer information about OCD without being self-conscious and thereby promotes a feeling of being understood. In this sense, the process of mapping OCD not only provides information for subsequent treatment, but also contributes to the child's hope and willingness to participate in treatment. By constructing the new story in this fashion, the child and therapist together no longer view OCD as an all-encompassing problem that is nearly synonymous with the child's life. Rather OCD becomes "enemy territory" that can be taken back through the techniques being taught in CBT.

At the conclusion of Session 3, the therapist and child should have agreed on a symptom hierarchy that includes all the important OCD symptoms that trouble or interfere with the child's life. During Session 4, the therapist and child will work toward a comprehensive view of which triggers on the hierarchy fall within the transition zone and are thus reasonable candidates for E/RP targets.

## LEARN TO USE REWARDS

OCD will not resolve with contingency management strategies such as those used for attention-deficit/hyperactivity disorder (ADHD). However, positive reinforcement can be quite helpful in increasing the motivation to resist OCD, especially for the child who has been exposed to a steady stream of verbal negativity or punishment because of OCD symptoms (whereas punishment almost invariably makes OCD worse). Rewards for successfully "bossing back OCD" in the form of verbal praise, small prizes, or minicertificates can be presented during and at the end of each treatment session. The child should also be told during Session 1 that a graduation diploma certifying that the child has successfully "beaten up" OCD will be presented at the conclusion of treatment. Rewarding each successful "bossing back" of OCD helps to remind the child concretely that he or she is the author of a new story in which OCD gradually becomes less bossy. Rewards for specific tasks also help the child continue to identify OCD as the problem, while increasing self-esteem and motivation. Lest parents think that this is bribery, we usually remind them that resisting OCD is hard work and might reasonably be rewarded just like any other chore. Since the motivational potency of rewards varies tremendously with the age of the child and the family culture within which the rewards occur, the therapist should individualize rewards based on what works for the individual child.

## DEVELOPMENTAL CONSIDERATIONS

As noted previously, therapists should adjust their level of discourse and the examples they use to the level of cognitive functioning, social maturity, and capacity for sustained attention of each child or adolescent participating in treatment. For example, cognitive training will need to be more concrete for younger patients, while, for example, there is more latitude for judgments about what is reasonable fastidiousness in mature adolescents. Similarly, the process of negotiating hierarchies requires greater initiative on the part of the therapist when the patient is younger or lacks good organizational skills. The therapist should be flexible and keep these developmental considerations in mind throughout all treatment sessions.

## PARENT CHECK-IN

As part of setting up the hierarchy, parents can be encouraged to identify triggers they may have observed to be part of OCD's territory. These may be observations about the child and OCD or about how OCD traps family members in rituals. The latter will be the focus of later sessions so that it is not critical to generate a detailed map of potential extinction targets now. The therapist should solicit information from parents in a gentle way, remembering that parent, therapist, and child are all on the same team to fight against OCD. Therapists should reframe parent comments, such as "Johnny always gets upset if we don't wash his silverware twice before dinner," which appear to blame the child instead of OCD. For example, this statement could be reworded as "So it sounds like OCD is bossing you and Johnny around by insisting on rewashing silverware. In this case, eating with silverware triggers OCD to create the worry that the silverware is contaminated and therefore must be washed, which is the compulsion. Does that sound right to you Johnny?" As in previous sessions, parents should also be encouraged to praise the child for resisting OCD, while at the same time refocusing their attention on positive elements in the child's life (DRO).

## EVALUATION

The therapist should spend a few minutes charting ratings on the NIMH Global OC Scale and the CGI scales.

## HOMEWORK

The homework given at Session 3 involves two types of tasks:

- First, to lay the groundwork for identifying the transition/work zone during the next session, the child should continue being a detective with OCD and should pay particular attention during the coming week to situations in which OCD wins some of the time and the child wins some of the time. It is sometimes helpful for the child to keep a notebook to record informal notes about each item on the symptom hierarchy. In this way, the child can check the accuracy of the hierarchy and gather information about how easy it is to engage in spontaneous E/RP.
- Second, while gathering information about items on the symptom hierarchy, the child should practice the short form of the cognitive tactics agreed upon during this session. Here again, the idea is not to suddenly cease participating in rituals, but rather to understand how well the cognitive interventions work, given the particulars of the child's OCD symptoms, so that these cognitive strategies can be refined for use during the E/RP tasks that will begin next week. A good place to examine the utility of the cognitive interventions is with unavoidable triggers for OCD symptoms that the child can often successfully resist.

# Chapter 7

## Session 4: Completing the Tool Kit

Carla has played detective again this past week and has spent more time watching for those situations when sometimes she wins and sometimes OCD wins. She realized, for example, that between her math and English classes, when she doesn't have time to wash her hands, she generally goes ahead and uses her English book despite her fears of contamination. Another transition zone trigger occurs in the bathroom with the sink handles. Carla noticed this week she was sometimes able to turn them off without using a paper towel. When she began to worry and felt like rewashing her hands, she was able to tell herself, "It's no big deal—just Germy trying to boss me," and left without the second washing. During this session, Carla decides to try this exposure task with Nadine. She reminds herself during the exposure task that the worry is just her brain playing tricks on her and that Germy isn't going to win this time. Carla uses the fear thermometer to measure her anxiety during the exposure task: it rises to a level 4–5 but within 20 minutes returns to a 1.

### GOALS OF SESSION 4

1. Finalize the transition zone.
2. Finalize the tool kit in preparation for E/RP.
3. Assign trial exposure tasks.

## REVIEW HOMEWORK

After checking on how things went in general, ask the child which OCD triggers he thinks belong in the transition/work zone (i.e., where the child is already successfully resisting OCD at least some of the time). For many youngsters, it is often helpful to break the transition zone into halves or even thirds, since E/RP targets should if possible be chosen from transition zone targets that the child already success-fully resists a majority of the time, at least at the beginning of treatment. The therapist should provide liberal positive reinforcement for the child's success in identifying and resisting OCD and should compliment the child for all successes, even if they are only partial. It is often a better strategy to reinforce feelings ("I bet that felt good") than to reinforce performance ("Good job, Billy"), especially in the child who tends to be self-critical.

If the child has not been able to make notes on the symptom list, the therapist may use this time to encourage the child to identify the transition zone while the therapist updates the list. Pay special atten-tion to how the child is feeling and coping in the ongoing battle with OCD and encourage the child to be patient while learning and practicing the strategies of CBT. Remind the child that you cannot play the piano expertly after only three lessons and that the same is true for CBT. Reinforce for the child that the therapist's role is that of a coach who will encourage and help the child find ways to succeed in completing E/RP tasks. The child's job is to practice the tools of CBT, so that OCD remits.

## FINALIZE THE TRANSITION ZONE

As each symptom or trigger on the map is identified and explored, the therapist and child use the fear thermometer to rate the child's anxiety level during a variety of hypothetical E/RP tasks. Lower levels of distress signal the location of the transition zone where OCD's terri-tory and the child's territory overlap. Because the child is more likely to accept and successfully complete an E/RP task chosen from the transition zone, this is the most effective place to initiate E/RP. Since some children find the terms transition or work zone difficult to understand, the therapist should be flexible in allowing the child to choose a label for this concept. While we call it the transition or work zone, children sometimes give it other names, such as TZ, or use a cartographic metaphor, such as Raleigh's place or Karen's office. If your patient has already chosen another name for the zone, you may continue using it; if not, it is fine to choose a name other than transition or work zone during this session. The important thing is again to emphasize the dual meanings of the transition zone (where OCD wins some of the time and the child wins some of the time) and the work zone (where the child will resist OCD by completing E/RP all the way to habituation).

The transition zone inevitably changes during treatment as the child claims back more and more territory from OCD (i.e., the transition zone moves up the stimulus hierarchy). Identifying where both OCD and the child compete for influence in specific functional domains, such as at school or when getting ready for school, is a good way to identify transition zone OC symptoms. Exposure in these areas is always to some degree unavoidable. Sensitive interviewing will reliably uncover areas of the child's life that are already free from OCD, including those that were once bossed by OCD but no longer are.

Using the stimulus hierarchy, identify candidates for E/RP that fall in the transition zone. You can start at the top and work down or at the bottom and work up. Since the symptom hierarchy is really a general tool, it may be helpful to break individual items down into steps that correspond to the transition zone for a particular OCD trigger. For example, it may not be possible to stop washing, but it may be okay not to do each finger in order. The process of "violating the rules" when doing rituals is further defined in Session 5, when E/RP begins in earnest. (If time permits, you may wish to introduce some of the concepts from Session 5 at this time.) Once the therapist and child have located the transition/work zone together, a trial exposure task can be selected from this zone.

## FINALIZE THE TOOL KIT

The child now has several tools to use in combating OCD: a mechanism for selecting E/RP targets from the transition zone, the fear thermometer, a variety of cognitive strategies, and rewards for efforts made to boss back OCD. Using the analogy to a doctor's bag or carpenter's belt may help some children better understand the idea of carrying a bag of coping strategies into battle with OCD. E/RP is the most powerful tool in the kit and must be chosen at the child's pace, using the transition zone, another tool. Coping strategies such as "talking back" to OCD, use of the fear thermometer throughout the exposure task, and rewards after exposure are tools that can be used or practiced apart from and during both imaginal and in vivo exposure tasks. Before conducting a trial exposure task, the therapist should remind the child of all the tools he or she has learned and rehearse the short form of the cognitive training approach agreed upon during the last session.

## ASSIGN TRIAL EXPOSURE TASKS

Before the session ends, practice a trial E/RP task to illustrate the points covered in this session and to show the child that it is indeed possible to successfully "beat up OCD." Be sure to help the youngster choose a task from the transition/work zone that will produce a level of anxiety that is low enough for the child to tolerate throughout the exposure task. The child can perform this therapist-assisted E/RP task imaginally or in vivo (i.e., he can imagine touching a "contaminated" door knob and not washing or he can really do it, assuming that an in vivo target is easily accessible in the office setting). During the task, the therapist helps the child use the fear thermometer by asking him to rate his or her anxiety at specified intervals (e.g., every 2 minutes during E/RP). In this way, we introduce the principle that anxiety will attenuate, rather than continue to rise, with prolonged exposure. The therapist may coach the child during the exposure task by "talking back" to OCD for the child. Before beginning a trial E/RP task, be sure that enough time is left in the session (usually 10 minutes is more than adequate for such an easy task) to move through exposure-based anxiety to habituation. Dialogue 7.1 illustrates how the therapist can introduce the notion of a trial exposure task:

*Dialogue 7.1*

NADINE: Let's try to boss back Germy right now.

CARLA: Sure, but how can I?

NADINE: Look at the map and pick out a situation when Germy tries to boss you around, but your fear thermometer does not go up very far. Use the transition zone to help you pick. For example, how far would your fear thermometer go up if you touched the sink in the bathroom without washing your hands?

CARLA: That would be too hard—it would go up to a 9 or 10.

NADINE: Okay, is there something you could touch that would only make your anxiety go up to a 4 or 5?

CARLA: I could touch just the handles on the sink.

NADINE: Great. Would you be willing to try that exposure task with my help?

CARLA: What will I have to do?

NADINE: We would go into the bathroom together and, when you touch the handles on the faucet, I will ask you how high your fear thermometer has gone up. Then, every 1–2 minutes I will ask you again how high your fear is until it has come all the way down to a level of 1 or 0. The most important part is that you not wash your hands or wipe them off in any way until your anxiety has come all the way down. Okay?

CARLA: Okay, I'll try.

## PARENT CHECK-IN

As in previous sessions, parents are encouraged to praise their child for resisting OCD, while at the same time refocusing their attention on positive elements in the child's life. The therapist should also address parents' concerns and questions and encourage their feedback on the child's progress.

## EVALUATION

The therapist should spend a few minutes charting ratings on the NIMH Global OC Scale and on the CGI scales.

## HOMEWORK

• This session's homework is to practice a trial exposure each day. From the therapist's point of view, the purpose of a trial exposure is to assess the accuracy of the stimulus hierarchy with respect to difficulty, ascertain compliance, and assess the child's ability to rate anxiety. The specific task chosen may be the one practiced during this session or another that the child feels more ready to do at home. In either case, the child should practice choosing the task from the transition/work zone. *Since failure will make future E/RP tougher to negotiate, the chosen task must be one that the child absolutely, positively can navigate successfully.* Because the therapist is not available to assist, the same task that produces a fear thermometer rating of 5 in the office may produce a rating of 8 at home. The therapist should therefore be especially cautious about letting the child proceed very far up the stimulus hierarchy; it is usually better to choose something "too easy." Children often do not tolerate anxiety well, particularly when surprised or ill-prepared, so prevention rather than "picking up the pieces" is by far the wiser course.

• Some E/RP tasks involve *choosing* to face a feared stimulus that could be avoided (termed *contrived exposure*); others involve preventing rituals in response to OCD triggers that cannot be avoided (called *uncontrived exposure*). If the selected task involves contrived exposure, a specific time for the homework task should be set aside each day. If response prevention (RP) in response to uncontrived exposure is chosen, designating a "window" for RP is acceptable, or the child can engage in RP at every instance of exposure to the trigger, depending on the particular circumstances.

• As modeled during the session, the child is instructed to rate his or her anxiety at 2–3 minute intervals throughout the exposure task, using the Homework Sheet provided in Appendix I (Handout 5) for this purpose.

• During the exposure task, the child is encouraged to "talk back" to OCD, especially when the urge to ritualize rises, and to refuse to ritualize until the fear thermometer comes down to a level of 1 or 2. The child should be encouraged to start using the short-form cognitive training rubric, including the 3" × 5" card prepared earlier for just this purpose, as soon as he or she begins to feel anticipatory anxiety when contemplating the approaching E/RP task.

# Chapter 8

# Session 5: Putting E/RP into Action

Carla has tried her sink handle exposure task almost every day over the past week. When asked how high her anxiety goes now when she turns the sink off without paper towels or extra washing, Carla replies it only goes to a 2 and sometimes she doesn't think about it at all. She reports feeling very encouraged and confident and wants to get on with "mushing OCD." During today's session, Carla is able to identify some new targets for the stimulus hierarchy that involve her parents. Her mother has to wash her sheets every day because Germy will give Carla anxiety later at night if they are not clean. Her mother also has to re-wash drinking glasses before giving Carla something to drink. Carla places these and a few other items on her hierarchy list and assigns a fear temperature for each if her mother does not do what Germy requires.

## GOALS OF SESSION 5

1. Identify OCD's influence with family members.
2. Continue imaginal and/or in vivo E/RP.

## REVIEW HOMEWORK

After checking on how things have gone in general, evaluate the outcome of the trial exposure task assigned during the last session with respect to motivation, accuracy of predicting anxiety levels, parental involvement, impact of comorbid conditions, or other obstacles. Treat last week's E/RP task as information rather than as a predictor of future success in E/RP. The purposes of trial E/RP tasks are to gather information and practice anxiety-reduction before E/RP begins in earnest during this session. A common misconception is that a trial exposure task should not produce anxiety; however, any E/RP produces definite anxiety, which the child must then tolerate. The central question in evaluating the trial exposure task is how much anxiety the child is presently able to tolerate. The therapist and child should have selected an exposure task that the child could complete without resorting to compulsions. If the child had considerable trouble with the trial exposure task, it may mean that that the location of the transition/work zone must be revised and that more detailed but simpler and more easily resisted E/RP targets should be chosen. Since children with OCD are always at risk of "bailing out" of E/RP homework, it is necessary to find tasks that the child can follow through with completely. Otherwise, the treatment itself ends up reinforcing OCD and compliance will plummet.

If the child consistently "bailed out" (e.g., used escape–avoidance maneuvers to handle anxiety) in the middle of the E/RP task, simply point out that the chosen task was clearly too difficult. It is good to know this at this point so that the child can choose an E/RP task that is more suitable. Alternatively, the therapist can discuss possible strategies the child might have used to ensure success. Since the task chosen was from the easy end of the transition/work zone, use the child's successful attempts to "boss back" OCD as much as possible to provide a solid "proof" that the child will, with practice, be able to write OCD out of his or her story.


## IDENTIFY OCD'S INFLUENCE WITH FAMILY MEMBERS

Parents, family members, and friends often end up participating in rituals and thus become entangled in OCD's territory. Much of the functional impairment and negativity associated with OCD arise because of the impact OCD has on other people besides the affected child. It is therefore critical to assess the extent to which OCD has involved other family members. (For a more detailed discussion of family involvement, see Chapters 10, 12, and 19.)

To maintain the therapist's position as the child's coach, it is wise to give the child an opportunity to report on how OCD tangles up all family members. Ask the child to talk a bit about how OCD bosses around his or her parents and to speculate about what the fear thermometer "temperature" would be if his or her parent(s) were to boss OCD back. OCD symptoms involving parents (and others, such as siblings and teachers) can then be positioned on the symptom hierarchy along with the corresponding rating or "temperature." Tell the child that, if ready to do so, he or she will have the opportunity to ask parents to stop participating in rituals during Sessions 7 and 12.

The therapist should also address other questions or concerns about the upcoming parent session with the child during this session.

## UPDATE SYMPTOM HIERARCHY

It is important to update the symptom hierarchy at each session to ratify the location of the child's transition/work zone and, if necessary, to add new or subtract old OCD symptoms. Updating the hierarchy also provides positive feedback to the child as he or she reclaims territory from OCD and sees how the transition zone moves up the symptom list. Ask the child to review the Symptom List and indicate if any fear thermometer "temperatures" have changed or if there are any new symptoms to add to the list.

## CONTINUE E/RP

By now the basic concept of choosing a new E/RP target from the symptom hierarchy, practicing an imaginal or in vivo E/RP task in the office, and setting up E/RP homework should be familiar to both child and therapist. Depending on the nature of the child's OCD symptoms, his or her cognitive abilities, and the support available from family and friends, it may be helpful to review all or some of the following points.

### Contrived versus Uncontrived Exposure

In *contrived exposure*, the child *chooses* to face a feared stimulus that could be avoided (i.e., it is the opposite of intentional avoidance).

Avoidance behaviors should have been placed on the stimulus hierarchy, so that, when ready, the child may chose a contrived exposure task in which he or she will *on purpose* seek out and stay in contact with a phobic object until habituation occurs. Preventing escape–avoidance (defined as bailing out in the middle of contrived exposure) is a response prevention (RP) procedure, with avoidance defined as a ritual in this case.

In *uncontrived exposure*, the child comes into contact with an OCD trigger that is essentially unavoidable, which usually results in the performance of rituals. The purpose of RP in uncontrived exposure is to prevent or modify the ritual.

In selecting E/RP targets for this week's homework, the child may do a contrived exposure task (i.e., seek out the trigger) or may just focus on RP in response to uncontrived exposure. Paying attention to the distinction between contrived exposure (ending avoidance) and uncontrived exposure (picking RP targets) may make it easier for the child to feel in control and, therefore, to make a successful choice of E/RP targets.

## Exposure for Obsessions and/or Mental Rituals

In addition to the cognitive therapy interventions detailed earlier (constructive self-talk, cognitive restructuring, and cultivating detachment), two other techniques may prove helpful to those children who have OCD symptoms that involve only thoughts.

First, it is sometimes useful to allocate a specific "worry time," say 10 minutes twice a day, that the child can devote to an obsession, while resisting it as usual at other times. This encourages the child to defer obsessing, which involves response prevention, and therefore encourages extinction of the OCD symptom. The "worry period" also provides an element of exposure. It is important that the child not think positive thoughts during the "worry period" and instead work to become as distressed as possible, by repeating the worry over and over again. This technique is sometimes called "satiation," and is discussed in more detail in Chapter 18.

Second, it is sometimes helpful to use a 1-minute closed-loop audiotape (as used in telephone answering machines). Ask the child to write down his or her obsessions verbatim as they enter the mind and then to record them on the audiotape in your presence, making the tone of his or her voice match the feelings that characterize the obsession as much as possible. Schedule a 30- to 45-minute session once a day during which the child listens to the audiotape over and over using a portable tape player with headphones, such as a Sony Walkman, and attempts to generate as much distress as possible.

When children use either of these interventions, they typically become distressed at the beginning, but are bored by the end of the prescribed homework period—which is just what is intended. Toward the end of the week, therefore, the procedure can be terminated if the initial SUDS scores fail to rise beyond negligible levels of anxiety. When the practice is no longer serving as an OCD trigger, it may be necessary to chose another worry for "worry time" or to substitute a different worry for use with the closed-loop audiotape. For most patients, however, it is best to do the procedure for a week without any change to avoid any possibility of escape–avoidance and to ensure habituation of the anxiety associated with the obsession.

Dialogue 8.1 illustrates how the therapist can introduce these techniques.

## Dialogue 8.1

NADINE: Carla, you've told me about some worry thoughts that pop into your head and stay there for a while.

CARLA: Yeah, like yesterday, when I couldn't stop trying to figure out if there will be a nuclear war.

NADINE: And when you had this thought, did anything trigger it?

CARLA: No, it just popped into my head.

NADINE: Well, I know another tool you can use to boss back this kind of worry thought. Would you like to try it?

CARLA: I don't know—what is it?

NADINE: Well, remember when we talked about how, after you've gone on a roller coaster five times in a row, it's not nearly so scary as the first time?

CARLA: Yes.

NADINE: We can do the same thing with these thoughts by having you listen to them over and over again on purpose.

CARLA: But that will be scary.

NADINE: Yes, you're right, at first it will be scary, but gradually it'll become easier—just like the roller coaster.

CARLA: How would it work?

NADINE: There are two ways to try this. One way is to choose a time each day to worry about your OCD thought on purpose for about 10 or 15 minutes. Your job would be to worry as much as possible for 10 minutes, then stop and go do something fun. Each day you could practice this and, after a while, that worry thought will start to get boring because you have thought it so much.

CARLA: What's the other way?

NADINE: You could write down your worry thoughts when you have them. Then you could record them on a tape and listen to them on your Walkman. You could schedule a time each day to listen to the recording for 30 minutes or so.

CARLA: Okay, I think I'd like to use a tape recorder.

NADINE: Great! When do you want to schedule your practices?

CARLA: Well, I want to relax and do some homework after school. I could listen to the tape after dinner.

## Breaking the Rules

After embarking on contrived or uncontrived exposure, the next step is RP, without which habituation will not occur. Here the trick is to find ways for the child to violate the "rule made by OCD." While the general idea in RP is to work with the child (using the transition zone) to select E/RP targets, it is often difficult to precisely define a homework assignment using only the stimulus hierarchy. Ideally, the child would simply choose not to ritualize. However, this is too vague to be useful—and the child would already have done so if he or she could. Being more precise in specifying the intervention helps to ensure that the child can successfully complete it.

Table 8.1 presents four techniques for "breaking the rules" that OCD specifies for rituals: delaying, shortening, changing, or slowing down the ritual. When these techniques are integrated with the concept of the transition/work zone, they give the therapist a precise mechanism for defining a within-item transition zone for each item at the lower end of the symptom hierarchy. Another alternative is to add

**TABLE 8.1.** Techniques for "Breaking the Rules" of OCD

| Method | Description | Example |
|---|---|---|
| Delay the ritual. | Postpone doing the ritual for longer and longer predefined periods of time until eventually you "wait it out." | Delay washing for 1 hour. |
| Shorten the ritual. | Do the ritual, but for increasingly shorter periods of time, until you no longer need to do it. | Wash for 10 rather than 15 minutes. |
| Do the ritual differently. | Change some aspect of the ritual in a way that breaks the rule. | Don't wash fingers in order. |
| Do the ritual slowly. | Instead of rushing through the ritual to get it done, do it slowly and carefully, paying attention to the details of the ritual. | Wash each finger once carefully rather than over and over again. |

a consequence to the ritual (e.g., doing 30 minutes of piano practice); however, this is less practical for children because it smacks of punishment rather than deterrence.

In each case, the proposed change in the ritual is incompatible with the tendency inherent in OCD to keep the ritual unchanged or to expand the ritual. Thus, when using these RP techniques alone or in combination, anxiety should rise and come down over time (i.e., habituate) in a predictable fashion as measured by SUDS scores. Most important, by adjusting the level of difficulty of the task up or down, the child and therapist have considerable latitude in designing E/RP tasks that are neither too hard nor too easy for the particular OCD symptom trigger. The more inventive you can be in designing RP tasks, involving the child in developing creative ways to break OCD's rules, the more likely that the child can complete the E/RP task successfully. Dialogue 8.2 illustrates how the therapist can introduce the concept of breaking OCD's rules.

## Dialogue 8.2

NADINE: Carla, you know how Germy makes you wash in a certain way sometimes?

CARLA: Yeah, I have to wash each finger separately starting with my thumb and going in order to my pinky. Then I have to wash the palms of my hands and, last, the tops.

NADINE: Well, how would you like to learn another way of bossing Germy so you aren't bothered by Germy when you wash?

CARLA: Okay.

NADINE: Since Germy is making you follow certain rules when you wash, one way to beat him is to break those rules. For example, you could wash in the opposite order or in a random way. When you do this, your fear thermometer will probably go up, but what do you think will happen to it after a little while?

CARLA: It will come back down, just like when I tried touching the door knob.

NADINE: That's right! And each time you break the rules, it will get easier and easier until eventually you won't even think about it. Would you like to try it with me?

CARLA: Okay, I'll give it a try.

NADINE: Before we start, are there any other rules that Germy makes you follow?

CARLA: Well, sometimes I have to walk around this one chair in a certain way. My grandmother used to sit in it when she was sick.

NADINE: Okay, let's put that on our Germy map. How high would your thermometer go if you broke the chair rule?

CARLA: That would be pretty hard—a 7 or 8, I think.

NADINE: How high do you think your thermometer will go when you break the washing rule?

CARLA: I think about a 4 or 5. It's in my T-zone a little already because sometimes I'm in a hurry and I don't do it.

NADINE: Great, let's give it a try.


Therapist-Assisted E/RP

The assistance of the therapist with E/RP in the office increases the likelihood that the child will succeed in the same task at home. It is helpful for the therapist to overtly model the exposure task (e.g., by touching a "contaminated" object). Covert modeling is also useful (e.g., the therapist does the exposure task without telling the child in advance or providing a rationale). This is clearly more practical for E/RP tasks for which the trigger is readily accessible in the office environment. Alternatively, the child's parent can sometimes bring an OCD trigger, such as a "contaminated" object, to the office. It may sometimes be necessary for the therapist to actually go to the home or school environment to support the child in successfully completing E/RP. Depending on the family circumstances, one or more family members can also be trained to function as a supportive cotherapist.

## DEVELOPMENTAL CONSIDERATIONS

The ability to tolerate exposure varies with age. Adolescents are usually able to tolerate a greater intensity of exposure than younger children, although at times the opposite is true. The ability to externalize or make OCD the problem also tends to vary between children and adolescents. Young children often have rituals that involve their families and may therefore see their rituals as part of everyday life. For example, a young girl who fears not wearing enough clothing to stay warm demands that her mother give her a weather report every day. The ritual of reporting the weather outside seems to be normal at first, but in fact it is part of OCD's territory. Some adolescents have difficulty externalizing OCD because OCD itself overlaps with identity issues. For example, a young man may question whether he is acting immorally when he experiences violent obsessions. Another common example of this involves the overlap between religious belief, culture-dependent homophobia, and OCD-related homophobia. In both examples, it is often difficult for the young person to tell himself that the obsession is simply OCD hiccuping away and has nothing to do with his own sense of morality. Without losing focus, it is important to explore these issues when setting up E/RP tasks. As noted previously, therapists should adjust the level of discourse and examples used to the level of cognitive functioning, social maturity, and capacity for sustained attention of each child or adolescent participating in treatment.

## PARENT CHECK-IN

Parents are encouraged to praise their child for resisting OCD and to continue DRO. The exceptionally supportive and sophisticated parent may be able to participate as a surrogate cotherapist for E/RP tasks at home.

## EVALUATION

The therapist should spend a few minutes charting ratings on the NIMH Global OC Scale and the CGI scales.

## HOMEWORK

The homework for the coming week involves daily practice of the exposure or response prevention task (or tasks) that the child has chosen from the transition/work zone.

• Be sure to pick a task that is "too easy" (e.g., one with which the child has already had considerable success). The duration of the exposure is not important as long as the child completes the task and sticks with it until his or her anxiety attenuates to a fear thermometer rating of 2 or less for several minutes. Telling the child to do it until it becomes boring is often sufficient advice. Reinforce the strategies discussed at the beginning of this session to ensure effective practice of the exposure task.

• Remind the child to use his or her preferred cognitive "tool kit" during E/RP and to measure and record anxiety levels at regular intervals using the fear thermometer.

Since E/RP has now begun in earnest, the therapist should schedule a between-session telephone call before the child leaves to see if the child is having any problems completing the homework task. If the child has chosen a task that has proved too difficult, the therapist can help the child modify the task, or less preferably, choose an alternate task over the telephone. If the child has forgotten to practice the E/RP task, the therapist can try to discover what obstacles are preventing the child from completing the homework practice. If the child has already habituated to this task (it indeed was "too easy"), the therapist and child can negotiate a more difficult E/RP task.

# Chapter 9

# Session 6: E/RP Continues

Carla comes to this session a little disappointed because she was unable to do the exposure task she chose last week. She contaminated her clothes on purpose at school, by leaning up against the lockers, but when she returned home, she was unable to keep from changing clothes and showering. As Nadine and Carla discuss what got in the way of the exposure task, Carla realizes she kept telling herself all day at school that she could always change clothes when she got home. Nadine helps Carla see that this thought is a type of compulsion (or mental ritual) that lets Germy win. During the session, they come up with a way to modify the exposure task so that Carla waits until the end of the school day to contaminate her clothes and then practices "talking back" to Germy on the way home.

## GOALS OF SESSION 6

1. Identify areas of difficulty with E/RP.
2. Continue therapist-assisted E/RP.

## REVIEW HOMEWORK

As always, check in about how things are going in the child's life. Evaluate the preceding week's E/RP task, paying particular attention to the child's anxiety ratings. Emphasize the process of habituation—that is, each time the child does the exposure task, his or her anxiety, as rated on the fear thermometer, will decrease more quickly and not rise as high.

## IDENTIFY AREAS OF DIFFICULTY

If the child is experiencing no change in anxiety ratings each time the task is performed, he or she may be using mental rituals that supersede or replace the previous compulsion. For example, some children turn OCD on its head by saying, "If I do the ritual, something bad will happen," thereby generating a new mental compulsion in place of the old ritual. Anxiety may also remain unchanged after several practice exposures if the child has not waited during the exposure task for his or her fear thermometer "temperature" to come down to a level of 1 or 0. Although dysphoric affects generally decrease within 20 or 30 minutes, it is not uncommon for anxiety to take up to an hour or more to abate. By rating anxiety at intervals throughout the exposure task, the child can ensure that he or she does not discontinue the exposure task before these feelings and the accompanying obsessions have receded. When anxiety remains high or, alternatively, fails to rise, the exposure task needs revision. The former is most often caused by the child "bailing out" before his or her anxiety attenuates, but may reflect an E/RP task that is simply too hard. Watch especially carefully when the chosen E/RP task no longer triggers anxiety, a new ritual is replacing the old one, or the child is managing anxiety using covert mental rituals. It is not uncommon to discover new rituals and triggers throughout treatment; a brief review of the symptom hierarchy is therefore essential at each visit. (A more detailed discussion of pitfalls in implementing E/RP is given in Chapters 17 and 18.)

Dialogue 9.1 illustrates how the therapist can address a situation in which anxiety remain high.

### Dialogue 9.1

CARLA: I tried to touch my dirty school books, but every time I did my anxiety just stayed up.

NADINE: It sounds like this task was quite hard for you. Let's see if we can figure out how Germy was able to win. How long were you able to hold your books?

CARLA: I held them for an hour, while I did my homework.

NADINE: What were you thinking about while you touched the books?

CARLA: I was thinking about all the people who had ever touched those books and how dirty they were. I told myself I could wash after I finished my homework.

NADINE: Okay, so while you were touching the books, it sounds like Germy was really bothering you with thoughts about the books and was reminding you to be sure to wash later. Did you have a chance to "talk back" to Germy?

CARLA: Well, no I didn't really. I just made sure I only touched the inside of the book.

NADINE: So Germy made you follow the "only touch the inside" rule, is that right?

CARLA: Yeah, I guess Germy was still bossing me around.

NADINE: Yes, I think Germy was, and that's why your thermometer would not come down. But now that we know how Germy kept you from the exposure task, we can figure out a game plan for getting Germy the next time. What did Germy make you do?

CARLA: Touch only the inside and think about all the germs.

NADINE: That's right. And Germy also reminded you to wash later, didn't he? Let's write down the tools you want to use to boss back Germy. First, touch all parts of the book, inside and out, and keep on touching all the parts. Second, use your thoughts to boss back Germy by reminding yourself that the anxiety will go away in a little while if you don't wash or even plan on washing. Another thought strategy is to talk back to those worry thoughts about germs. What could you tell yourself about that Germy book?

CARLA: I could say it's not that dirty, it's just Germy trying to bother me.

NADINE: That's right. Do you want to try again this week, now that you have a new game plan?

CARLA: Yeah, I'll be the boss this week.

NADINE: How about giving it a try right now in the office?
CARLA: Okay.

## CONTINUE THERAPIST-ASSISTED E/RP

In the office, the child rehearses those E/RP tasks that will be practiced at home and also tries E/RP tasks that are as yet too difficult to do at home. Once the child has succeeded imaginally or in vivo with the therapist, it will then be easier to choose more challenging exposure tasks for future homework. The child will also find it easier to accept challenging tasks if he or she is rewarded for any gains made, even if they are only partially successful. The therapist should stress the need to practice E/RP daily, using all the tools in the tool box.

## PARENT CHECK-IN

Parents are encouraged to continue DRO and positive reinforcement for resisting OCD. In anticipation of the next session (which is the first scheduled family session), parents are asked to think about the way OCD entangles family members.

## EVALUATION

During this session, the therapist should chart ratings on the NIMH Global OC Scale and on the CGI scales, and may wish to administer the YBOCS.

## HOMEWORK

• Ask the child to choose an exposure task from the transition zone to practice each day during the next week. Compliance can be enhanced by instructing the child to practice the homework task in the office in order to anticipate and correct potential problems. It may also improve compliance if the child sets aside a specific time to do the exposure homework. If he child is only willing or able to practice four times a week, homework assignments should be adjusted so that the child is not partially defeated before he or she begins. Response prevention when exposed to unavoidable targets (i.e., resisting OCD in the face of uncontrived exposure) should by now also have become a routine part of daily E/RP practice.

Again, the therapist should plan a midweek phone call to encourage the child in the E/RP task and to assess the need to modify the E/RP plan.

# Chapter 10

## Session 7: Family Session I

Carla's parents are pleased to see that Carla's hands are less chapped because she is washing less and Mom has noticed she even buys less soap now. Both parents, however, are still concerned with the many things they have to do in order to accommodate Germy. They also wonder sometimes if some of Carla's habits actually represent misbehavior. Nadine reviews with them the neurobehavioral framework for understanding OCD. Nadine also helps Carla's parents develop a hierarchy of ways in which Germy bosses around family members. She also encourages Carla's parents to talk about where they see Carla winning with OCD. They have already begun to reward Carla for her hard work completing exposure tasks each week by taking her out for ice cream after each session. Carla would like to have a pizza party when she's finished bossing back Germy and her parents are eager to help plan for one.

### GOALS OF SESSION 7

1. Include parents in treatment.
2. Plan ceremonies and notifications.
3. Continue E/RP.

## REVIEW HOMEWORK

As always, check in about how things are going in the child's life. Evaluate the preceding week's E/RP task, paying particular attention to whether the task lead to satisfactory habituation (as measured on the fear thermometer) so that this task can be considered completed. Revise the stimulus hierarchy as necessary.

## BACKGROUND FOR PARENT SESSION

While family dysfunction does not cause OCD, families nonetheless affect and are affected by the child with OCD. Moreover, OCD is substantially heritable. Twenty percent of affected children have an affected first-degree relative; many others have a family member with either an internalizing disorder or Tourette syndrome. Parents (both with and without symptoms) frequently become entangled in the child's rituals in order to reduce the child's and their own discomfort. Other parental concerns include control struggles surrounding rituals, difficulty dealing with sexual or aggressive obsessions, and differences of opinion about how to deal with OCD symptoms. Adolescents occasionally find rituals an effective weapon in the struggle for separation and can be reluctant to give them up, even when OCD itself interferes with individuation. In addition, OCD typically unsettles the family's social and community interactions, including those with health care professionals who may or may not understand the disorder. It is therefore crucial to understand the extent to which family members are tangled up in OCD, the capacity of the family to be supportive of the affected child, and conversely, the extent to which family psychopathology interferes with the implementation of CBT.

Chapter 19 ("Working with Families") provides essential background for the interventions discussed below. As Chapter 19 illustrates, the complexity of the interventions called for by variations in family functioning are impossible to address completely in this manual. Thus, clinical judgment and expertise come into play in dealing with families perhaps more than in any other situation, with the possible exception of handling complex comorbid conditions. For the purpose of discussion, however, we assume here that we are treating an average child with OCD, which calls for involving parents in some but not all sessions.

## INCLUDE PARENTS IN TREATMENT

Depending on the family's situation, the therapist may decide to hold all or part of this session with both parents and child present, or with child or parents alone. When siblings are also tangled up in OCD, including them in the sessions is also appropriate, depending on the objective for the session. For example, when sibling issues concerning OCD are paramount and/or are lower on the hierarchy as targets for E/RP than parent extinction tasks, then including siblings is warranted. When parental extinction tasks are urgently needed, including siblings makes sense in two circumstances: (1) if a sibling is especially supportive of the youngster with OCD or (2) if your patient's siblings are punitive in a way that interferes with the implementation of OCD. In the latter situation, working with all family members, including siblings, to minimize negative emotions concerning OCD or other family issues may be one key to moving treatment for OCD forward, so that including everyone at this session becomes necessary.

### The Purpose of Treatment

We begin by reviewing the neurobehavioral framework for OCD in the context of the overall treatment plan, paying special attention to the concept of E/RP. It is important to distinguish between "graded" E/RP that is under the child's control and a "just say no to OCD" approach, which most parents and children will already have tried without success. It is also helpful to review what went poorly in previous attempts at treatment and to ascertain parents' opinions of the current treatment. In discussing these topics with parents, the therapist should use externalizing language to reinforce the idea that parents and therapist alike are allies in the child's efforts to write OCD out of his or her story. Approaching parents in this fashion helps keep the focus on OCD as the problem and discourages blaming either the child or the parent(s) for continued OCD symptoms.

### The Role of Parents in Treatment

Despite being angry, confused, or frightened at times, parents are almost always consciously supportive of the child with OCD; however, parents also just as often find themselves unwittingly supporting OCD. In order for the child to make progress against OCD, parents must disengage from OCD and become wholly supportive of the child. To do so, it is imperative that the therapist continue to "make OCD the problem" in the narrative of this session, and not allow blaming and fault finding to emerge between family members. Parents can play one of several roles with respect to OCD:

- Helper of OCD: a nontherapeutic role that needs to be written out of the child's story.
- Cheerleader for the child.
- Cotherapist (almost always with the child's permission).

Obviously, we want to discourage the first, encourage the second, and carefully structure the third. These terms, which you may or may not want to use, are less important than the concepts, which imply that the therapist transfers control over OCD via skill building to the child directly and, directly or indirectly, to the parent. Not surprisingly, implementing parental behavior change in a way that keeps everyone—child, parent, and therapist—successfully aligned against OCD is not easy. For example, a parent who ceases to provide reassurance about a contamination fear is generating a response prevention task for the child. Thus, all changes in parental behavior relative to OCD must first be screened for their location on the stimulus hierarchy and implemented, if possible, with the child's assent. Dialogue 10.1 illustrates how the therapist can introduce parents to the different roles they can play in relation to OCD.

## Dialogue 10.1

NADINE: Thank you for coming today. These parent sessions are an opportunity for you to ask more questions about the treatment as well as a time to provide you with some tools for helping Carla with her OCD.

MOM: We're very interested in learning what we can do to help.

DAD: Yes, we'd like to do whatever we can.

NADINE: There are several different roles a parent can play with a child who has OCD. Often parents help OCD without realizing it. This happens when OCD makes you do things, like buying extra paper towels or washing extra laundry.

MOM: I have to wash my hands before I hand Carla a plate of food.

NADINE: That's a good example. One of the things we will want to do today is to map out all the things you have to do for Carla's OCD. We want to eventually eliminate your role as OCD's helper.

DAD: But what can we do?

NADINE: The most helpful thing you can do, especially in the beginning of treatment, is to be Carla's cheerleader. You can encourage Carla as she chooses E/RP tasks by letting her know you know how hard she is working. Another way of cheerleading is to pay lots of attention to those areas of Carla's life that are going well, such as her swimming. One of the best ways to help Carla fight OCD is to decrease the attention it gets.

MOM: Should I ask her about her E/RP homework?

NADINE: You might ask about it briefly once between sessions, but on the whole it is usually best to leave the homework up to Carla. Too much pressure about E/RP tasks can create an atmosphere of anxiety which, in turn, can increase their difficulty.

DAD: You said there was another role we could play?

NADINE: Yes—the role of cotherapist. Usually parents don't play the role of cotherapists until a little later in treatment. You have already begun, however, when you helped Carla eat the "contaminated" cookie which you dropped on the floor.

MOM: Yes, she practiced that one several times, and it did get easier. Now she can eat a snack without having to wash her hands for 5 minutes beforehand.

NADINE: Another way to be a cotherapist will occur when Carla gives you permission to stop doing the activities you now do for OCD, such as washing your hands before handing her a plate of food.

DAD: Should we start doing that anyway?

NADINE: It depends on Carla, and how much anxiety she will experience if you stop various OCD activities. We like to have the child choose when parents will stop, so that there are no surprises for the child and anxiety can be better managed. If, however, there are some tasks you feel you could stop doing without Carla becoming too upset, then we may want to give those a try. It would be helpful to ask Carla first. If Carla is not ready for you to stop certain activities, then it's best to stay in the role of cheerleader.

Very simply, we involve parents in the treatment process by helping the parents (or siblings) and child decide *together* how the parents (or siblings) will no longer participate in OCD. The child must choose targets in which family members stop participating in rituals. Because blocking rituals or avoidance behaviors removes the negative reinforcement effect of the rituals or avoidance, response prevention technically is an extinction procedure. However, extinction is more commonly referred to in clinical circles as the elimination of OCD-related behaviors through removal of parental positive reinforcement. Whatever term or definition you choose, parents must withdraw from rituals in a way that is manageable for the child. For example, a parent who is repeatedly washing dinner glasses before dinner until they are "clean enough" might, with the child's permission, cut down or eliminate this washing ritual. To make this happen, the therapist provides specific coaching for family members who will be participating in these E/RP tasks. Dialogue 10.2 illustrates how the therapist can help the child and parents choose appropriate targets for extinction.

## Dialogue 10.2

NADINE: Let's ask Carla if she would like you to choose a target for response prevention. Carla, your mom and dad have been telling me a little about how Germy bosses them around.

CARLA: What do you mean?

NADINE: Well, sometimes Germy makes them do some extra washing too, like before setting food on the table.

MOM: Yes, and you know how many towels we go through in a week.

NADINE: Just like we mapped out all the ways Germy bothers you, Carla, your parents and I mapped out some of the ways Germy bothers them. But we need your help to decide how your parents can start ignoring Germy.

CARLA: Okay. What do I do?

NADINE: Here's the list your parents made. Let's use the fear thermometer to rate how high your anxiety would go if they stopped doing these things.

CARLA: Well, if they stopped washing before setting the food on the table, that would be a 3 or 4 because sometimes I don't care if they wash.

NADINE: Okay, it sounds like that one belongs in the transition zone.

MOM: What if I didn't wash your sheets every night?

CARLA: That would be harder—I think it would be a 7.

NADINE: Carla, you've done a good job of rating each of these. Which one would you like your parents to stop doing first?

CARLA: Well, I'm not too sure. How about the washing at dinner?

NADINE: Okay, how does that sound to you, Mrs. Bailey?

MOM: It sounds great! Are you sure, Carla?

CARLA: Yes, I'm sure. I don't want Germy to boss you around, too.

Parents often wish to stop participating in certain rituals despite the fact that doing so would cause great distress in the child that the parents might be unable to manage. When family members are "sick of OCD," the slightest improvement can sometimes result in intolerable pressure to get better quickly. When the demand for the child to "improve" is strong, the therapist must counsel patience on the part of the parents, using the stimulus hierarchy to demonstrate that some tasks—no matter how burdensome OCD might be—are for the moment impossible. Stated differently, the therapist needs to help parents understand the importance of moving up the symptom hierarchy at the child's pace, letting the child choose how to withdraw parents from the role of OCD's "helper" so that they can assume the role of "cheerleader" or "cotherapist/coach."

Before parents begin to play the role of cotherapist/coach, they typically assume the role of "cheerleader." This involves providing support and encouragement for the child as he or she practices bossing back OCD, and assumes that inappropriate giving of advice has given way to a commitment to the structure of CBT. Just as cheerleaders cheer the play at hand, so parents are taught to encourage their child in the exposure task at hand. This safeguards against general unhelpful encouragement to fight all of OCD all the time. Such focused encouragement should also include rewards that are contingently targeted to the child's actual efforts to resist OCD, as defined by the therapist and child during treatment sessions.

Once parents are accustomed to the structure of CBT, are comfortable with DRO, and have assumed the role of cheerleader, knowledgeable parents, with the child's assent, may become extensions of the therapist. In particular, at the child's request, parents may act as a coach during E/RP tasks, taking the child to exposure targets and assisting with response prevention. For example, the child may ask the parent to help keep the water turned off while the child is performing a contamination-related exposure task. Since acting as coach is a complex endeavor that is fraught with potential landmines inherent in the parent/child relationship, it should be undertaken only when conditions of kindness and mutual reciprocity prevail. Even then, it is important to formulate the parent coaching role in a way that allows the therapist to retain control of the structure of the treatment. This is accomplished primarily by having the therapist and child retain control over the selection of E/RP targets during the treatment sessions.

## Unilateral Extinction Procedures

Very rarely, when parents are enormously inconvenienced and the child is reluctant to resist OCD at all, or only resists minimally, it is reasonable to suggest that parents pick an extinction target without the child's consent. However, such unilateral extinction procedures have significant disadvantages, making them a treatment of last resort. These disadvantages include: (1) parents' lack of a workable strategy for managing the child's distress; (2) disruption of the treatment relationship; (3) parents' inability to target symptoms that are out-of-sight of parents and teachers; and, most importantly; (4) the failure of nonconsensual extinction to help the child internalize a more skillful strategy for coping with current and possible future OCD symptoms.

Note that the use of unilateral extinction contradicts the agreement with the child about how therapy will proceed. Therefore it is critical to construe parent-initiated extinction strategies as *separate* from the E/RP plan. Here it is often useful to suggest that they fall under parental prerogatives to make decisions about practical necessities of home life. For example, the parents may require that the child vacate the bathroom if someone else has to use it, regardless of whether the child has "finished" washing and irrespective of the position of this OCD target on the stimulus hierarchy. When an extinction procedure is selected out of necessity without the child's consent, it is crucial to help parents develop a strategy for managing both their own and the child's resultant distress. In this situation, both parents and child will need to be in the room during therapy more than is usual, since check-in with parents will take longer and parents will require greater support with homework assignments. Attention must be paid to reducing parents' advice, criticism, or other negative remarks, which sap the child's will to resist OCD for consensual E/RP targets. The therapist should also make sure the child understands the nature of and rationale for the extinction procedure before it happens.

## Family Therapy

In rare situations, extensive family work is required before parents and siblings can be disentangled from OCD. However, formal family therapy or marital counseling should be recommended as part of the child's treatment if (and only if) family dysfunction or marital discord are interfering with effective treatment of the child's OCD.

## PLAN CEREMONIES AND NOTIFICATIONS

Punishment is a sure way to take the wind out of the child's sails when the time comes to resist OCD. Positive reinforcement has the opposite effect—ceremonies and notification help the child write OCD out of his or her story. *Ceremonies* are special occasions that recognize the child's success in reducing the territory held by OCD. Ceremonies can be simple, such as just going out for pizza, or more complicated, as in having a get together with family or friends in which special mention of the child's progress is made. *Notification* includes letters or telephone calls that inform significant others, who might otherwise remain in the dark, about the child's progress. Ceremonies and notification are especially important when other people see the child only in terms of psychopathology or are blind to the child's progress. During this parent session, the therapist should gather ideas for ceremonies and notifications that are meaningful for the child.

## DEVELOPMENTAL CONSIDERATIONS

The extent of parental involvement depends in part on the developmental stage of the child. Very young children typically require more help from parents. Youngsters grappling with separation–individuation themes may have more difficulty accepting help from well-intentioned parents. In every case, the therapist should consider issues of social and cognitive maturity, as well as developmental imperatives, when structuring parental involvement in treatment.

## EVALUATION

The therapist should spend a few minutes charting ratings on the NIMH Global OC Scale and the CGI scales.

## HOMEWORK

• Toward the end of this session, the child chooses a new E/RP task or tasks for the coming week. If the child is not yet ready for a new task, he or she may continue practicing the task or tasks from last week. By this time, it is usual for the child to choose more than one task, with the therapist helping to structure a blend of contrived E/RP tasks and RP following uncontrived exposure.

• Depending on the extent to which parents are entangled in the child's rituals, a homework assignment for the parents may have emerged from the preceding discussion. This will usually involve an extinction task in which the parents, with the child's consent, refrain from participating in a ritual. To the extent that this poses a significant leap forward, it may be wise to minimize other E/RP homework until after the midweek phone call with the therapist.

• As noted above, parents may assume the role of cotherapist with the child's encouragement, although in some cases parents may independently change their behavior with the therapist's approval.

• During Session 12, parents will have another opportunity for parents to choose E/RP tasks. In the meantime, ask parents to watch for new or previously unidentified ways in which they may be reinforcing OCD. By working with the child, these can often be incorporated into homework assignments as treatment progresses so that, where appropriate, extinction tasks may now be blended in with other E/RP tasks at all upcoming sessions.

• The therapist should plan a midweek phone call to encourage the child in the E/RP task and assess the need to modify the E/RP program.

• Decide on ceremonies and appropriate notifications with parents and child. Set a goal for the first ceremony.

Chapter 11

# Sessions 8–11: Moving Up the Stimulus Hierarchy

Carla has successfully negotiated a number of E/RP tasks on the lower end of the symptom hierarchy; her symptom hierarchy has therefore gotten shorter each week as the transition/work zone has moved up the hierarchy. Carla prefers that her friends not know about Germy, but she did tell her grandmother about how much progress she has made and they went to the movies to celebrate. However, Carla is concerned about a problem she's been having at school. Her teacher has assigned class presentations, which are due in 2 weeks. Carla has begun to feel quite nervous about this—she is certain she will not be able to stand in front of the class to give her report. She asks Nadine if this could be OCD. Nadine explains to Carla that, while the anxiety may be similar, her symptoms are related to something called social anxiety. Carla decides to call social anxiety "Jitter" and she and Nadine decide on some ways to boss back Jitter. In the meantime, Carla decides to keep on working on some of the exposure targets that have not yet come all the way down to a level 1. In this way, she will have a little more energy to tackle Jitter.

## GOALS OF SESSIONS 8–11

1. Arrange rewards, ceremonies, and notifications.
2. Address comorbidity and therapy needs.
3. Continue therapist-assisted E/RP.

## REVIEW HOMEWORK

As always, the therapist should carefully review the homework. It is not unusual for a child to need frequent revision of homework assignments. If a child is having particular difficulty with homework, the therapist should increase opportunities for E/RP tasks during the session. These can be done imaginally or in vivo and may include "field trips" to facilitate the exposure task.

## ARRANGE REWARDS, CEREMONIES, AND NOTIFICATIONS

While children cannot be "bribed" out of OCD, concrete rewards and ceremonies can play an important part in successful treatment. Although relief from OCD symptoms is often reward enough for many children with OCD, ceremonies reinforce the fact that the child has taken back territory that no longer belongs to OCD. In addition to verbal praise and a small reward, we sometimes present certificates of achievement, which the child is encouraged to share ("notify") with close friends or family members. Of course, rewards, praise, and encouragement are also given along the way to facilitate the child's continued work toward each larger goal or stage. Such rewards and ceremonies are particularly important for children with comorbid conditions, who may feel easily overwhelmed by their problems and neglect to acknowledge the very real progress they have made.

The therapist, parent, and child should together determine the accomplishments (or the amount of territory conquered) necessary for a ceremony marking a new stage in treatment. Dialogue 11.1 illustrates how the therapist can help parents and child plan a ceremony.

### Dialogue 11.1

NADINE: Carla, you've done so well, I think it's time for a party!

CARLA: Cool! Mom and I were talking about going for ice cream with my friend, Kathy.

MOM: Her Dad and I are so proud of Carla, and also so grateful to you for helping her get rid of OCD. She deserves to have her successes recognized.

NADINE: Carla's done beautifully, but we still have a ways to go.

However, I think that she deserves a celebration for all the good work she's done so far. Carla, who would you like to invite?

CARLA: Kathy. She and I used to be good friends, but, with OCD, I stopped going to her house. Now that I don't have to worry about the bathroom anymore, I'd like to play with her again.

NADINE: Great, we can work on how to talk to Kathy about OCD if you'd like.


## ADDRESS COMORBIDITY AND THERAPY NEEDS

As we discussed in Chapters 1 and 2, OCD is commonly comorbid with other disorders, each of which involves its own set of problems that may or may not interact with OCD. The task of setting up a treatment program is a little like solving a game of pick-up sticks. Each stick is a potential treatment target—the trick is to identify all the sticks and correctly decide in what order to pick them up. For example, the child who cannot use the bathroom when anyone else is present because of social phobia, but needs to do an E/RP task for contamination fears in the bathroom, must first habituate to using the bathroom before proceeding to E/RP for OCD.

Comorbid treatment targets should be externalized rather than fused with OCD, so that treatment can be tailored to the specific problems that affect the child. This is particularly important in the case of depression, since CBT itself may be compromised because of the child's mood disorder. In this situation, it is usually wise to start treatment with a serotonin reuptake inhibitor. Once the mood disturbance is under control, CBT for OCD can be implemented along with cognitive therapy for depression. Similarly, disruptive behavior disorders (e.g., ADHD) always require treatment before OCD can be addressed with CBT, since oppositional behavior throws a monkey wrench into the child's ability to cooperate with CBT. In this instance, treating ADHD with a psychostimulant and initiating parent training are prerequisites for beginning CBT for OCD. The parent training will need to be carefully coordinated with respect to treatment for OCD, however, so that contingency management strategies (rewards and punishment) are not inappropriately applied to disruptive behaviors that are due to OCD rituals. For example, the 9-year-old boy who can only turn right—his obsession is that his father will die if he turns left—should be treated sympathetically and not dragged through the supermarket. Conversely, there is no reason (unless hoarding or other OCD symptoms interfere) that this child should not have a star chart that includes a reinforcement schedule for picking up his room and other household chores.

While it is beyond the scope of this book to address the treatment of comorbidity in detail, specific interventions, such as relaxation training and habit reversal, that can be applied to OCD as well as to complicating comorbid conditions are addressed in Chapter 18 ("Special Wrinkles"). Appendix III also contains references to the literature on comorbid conditions. After carefully identifying complicating comorbid conditions, the therapist should tailor treatment to include interventions for these conditions, mixing and matching components from different sources as needed. The addition of treatment modules beyond those required for OCD is, of course, likely to prolong treatment beyond the customary 12 to 20 sessions.

## CONTINUE THERAPIST-ASSISTED E/RP

In the office, the child rehearses those E/RP tasks that will be practiced at home and also tries E/RP tasks that are as yet too difficult to do at home. Once the child has succeeded imaginally or in vivo with the therapist, it will then be easier to choose more challenging exposure tasks for future homework. The child will also find it easier to accept challenging tasks if he or she is rewarded for any gains made, even if they are only partially successful. The therapist should stress the need to practice E/RP daily, using all the tools in the tool box.

## DEVELOPMENTAL CONSIDERATIONS

The ceremonies and notifications selected will depend partly on the nature of the child's social relationships, which in turn depend on his or her developmental stage. It is important to follow the child's lead in deciding what is meaningful or salient as a reward.

Comorbidity also varies with developmental stage. For example, separation anxiety is more common in younger children, while panic disorder is more common in adolescents. In the same way, selective mutism is more common in younger children, while social phobia is more common in adolescents. Both sets of disorders may share an underlying pathogenetic mechanism, with the symptomatic expression colored by the age of the child.

## PARENT CHECK-IN

Parents should now be involved in treatment at a level that reflects the needs of the child and family system.

## EVALUATION

During each session, the therapist should spend a few minutes charting ratings on the NIMH Global OC Scale and on the CGI scales. Ratings on the YBOCS should also be obtained around the eighth week of treatment (generally at Session 10).

## HOMEWORK

- Negotiate E/RP task or tasks to be practiced each week. Reinforce the idea that daily practice is more effective than sporadic trials.
- As appropriate, involve the parents in mutually consensual extinction strategies.
- Remind the child to use the "tool kit" when anxiety is difficult to manage and to continue the task until his or her anxiety has abated, even if this should take as much as an hour.
- Record both the assignment and reminders on the homework sheet to facilitate consistent compliance.

The therapist should schedule a midweek phone call to encourage the child in the E/RP task(s) and assess the need to modify the E/RP program.

# Chapter 12

# Session 12:
# Family Session II

Carla's parents have come for another family session. Since the last meeting, they have tried, with Carla's prior agreement, to stop doing some of the things Germy demanded, such as washing the sheets every day. When Carla asked if her sheets were washed, her mother calmly replied she would not be able to wash them that day, but if Carla wanted to try she would be welcome. When Carla protested, her mother lovingly reminded her of their agreement with Nadine and, after about 15 minutes, Carla was fine and used her "Germy" sheets. Mom says that Carla no longer asks about the sheets. Dad noticed that if they respond in a neutral but supportive way when Carla is obsessing about something, she is better able to avoid performing the compulsion. They feel ready to decide together with Carla on additional E/RP tasks. Carla agrees, and they choose to work on Carla's reassurance seeking. Carla gives Mom and Dad permission not to answer her questions about germs, but instead to gently remind her that they too are bossing back Germy.

## GOALS OF SESSION 12

1. Remap how OCD involves significant others.
2. Implement extinction tasks.
3. Continue E/RP.

## REVIEW HOMEWORK

This entire session is conducted with both parents and child present. After a brief check-in and review of the preceding week's homework, the child, parents, and therapist together begin by summarizing the child's progress in bossing back OCD. We especially encourage parents to speak positively about those areas in their child's life that are now free of OCD. However, we must also add a caution about parental praise. When praise is excessive or exaggerated, the child may feel pressured or threatened, especially since progress may have slowed down a bit as the child approaches the upper end of the stimulus hierarchy. Since performance anxiety can lead to resistance to new E/RP tasks, parents should be encouraged to make praise accurate, specific, and short. Conversely, some parents find it difficult to focus on the gains the child has made against OCD. Such parents may be frustrated with the territory OCD continues to control, especially when OCD seriously inconveniences family members. In such cases, parents should be encouraged to be realistic about what has been accomplished, while acknowledging that there is much left to do in the way of E/RP. Since many parents come to treatment with the idea of a rapid cure uppermost in their minds, it is often useful to explain that, while most children experience moderate to marked improvement with time, far fewer are cured. Thus, patience, kindness, and commitment to treatment are the best strategies for ensuring continued improvement. Dialogue 12.1 illustrates how the therapist can explain the concept of specific praise to parents.

### Dialogue 12.1

NADINE: One of the ways you can both be cheerleaders for Carla is by briefly praising those areas of OCD where Carla has regained control. It is important that the praise be specific and fairly brief so that Carla does not begin to become anxious about pleasing you.

MOM: What do you mean by specific?

NADINE: When you are specific in praise, you name the advantage, feeling, or strategy used in accomplishing the task you are pleased with. For example, when Carla has more time in the morning before school because she no longer has to do extra washing, your specific praise might be "Carla, I bet it feels good to have time to watch cartoons before school since you've been bossing back Germy."

DAD: What about the times when she *doesn't* boss back Germy?

NADINE: It is very difficult, if not impossible, to get rid of all Carla's symptoms at one time, so usually it is more encouraging for Carla if you pay attention to the ways she is winning rather than focusing on symptoms that are still difficult. It's much like cheerleading for Carla when she plays soccer. During the game, you cheer when her team makes a good play or scores a goal, but what do you do when the other team makes a goal?

DAD: Nothing, except groan a little inside.

NADINE: It's the same with Germy—it may feel bad when Germy wins a play, but the less attention Germy gets for making the "goal," the better.

## REMAP OCD

To understand in detail how OCD entangles family members, we ask parents and child to consider together how OCD still influences their lives, that is, to remap OCD's territory in present time. At this point in treatment, parents will probably be able to see areas where OCD no longer tries to influence them, because the child has reclaimed that territory. There may be other areas where the parents cannot imagine responding differently for fear of their son or daughter's reaction. By carefully reconfirming the transition/work zone and examining it for the presence of extinction targets, the therapist can establish E/RP targets that include disentangling family members from OCD. To do so, parents and child must agree on which tasks would produce unmanageable anxiety and which would be more easily managed. The former must be postponed; the latter are targets for E/RP and parental extinction strategies.

## IMPLEMENT EXTINCTION TASKS AND CONTINUE E/RP

With the stimulus hierarchy remapped, it is now possible to negotiate consensual selection of E/RP (or extinction) targets from the transition/work zone. For example, if OCD requires a parent to rewash dishes before eating and the parent has decided, with the child's permission, to stop rewashing, then the child will need to use cognitive techniques to handle his or her anxiety. The parent reinforces the child in the use of such strategies during E/RP and so acts as cotherapist during the exposure task. Ask parents and child to imagine what is likely to happen when the parents respond to OCD in this new way. Troubleshoot reactions that may lead to "bailing out" (avoidance) of the task. Practice strategies for handling these specific behaviors. A simple reminder to the child of the agreements made during this session and encouragement to use his or her "tool kit" may be all that is needed to manage peak anxiety and then to proceed with the E/RP task until anxiety abates.

At the child's request, parents who are not entangled in OCD may still act as cotherapists for the child during the chosen exposure tasks. When parents are especially savvy with respect to the co-therapy role, the therapist at this juncture may feel very comfortable in transferring control for modifying and even, in some cases, choosing E/RP tasks during the coming week from the therapist to the parent(s). For this to happen, the parents should have read widely about the treatment of OCD and the relationship between the parent and child should be largely free from other than ordinary conflict.

## DEVELOPMENTAL CONSIDERATIONS

Some older children and adolescents may wish to assume full responsibility for doing their own E/RP tasks in a way that allows them to fulfill their developmentally normal need for autonomy. As long as CBT for OCD is going well, such needs should be honored. However, when the need for autonomy is interfering with successful CBT, the therapist should directly address the conflict between parents and child or adolescent during treatment.

## EVALUATION

The therapist should spend a few minutes charting ratings on the NIMH Global OC Scale and on the CGI scales.

## HOMEWORK

• In addition to choosing an extinction procedure with his or her parents, the child may also choose a new E/RP task to practice this week. If the parents' task will be particularly challenging, the child may continue practicing the exposure task from the previous week and/or focus on coping with the anxiety that results when the parents boss back OCD.

The therapist should schedule a midweek phone call to encourage the child in the E/RP task and assess the need to modify the E/RP program.

Chapter 13

# Sessions 13–18: Completing E/RP

Carla is excited as she comes into the office because she has been able to touch the inside of the bathroom sink at school without washing her hands. Her counting rituals also no longer bother her and, as she looks at her symptom hierarchy, there are only four more items to tackle. Carla also has given her parents permission to stop doing extra washing. Reassurance seeking is much reduced; inappropriate reassurance giving is negligible. Her mother let Carla buy something special with the money they saved this month from not buying so many bars of soap and paper towels.

## GOALS OF SESSIONS 13–18

1. Review child's overall progress.
2. Address plateaus.
3. Choose harder E/RP tasks.
4. Select parents' E/RP targets.

## REVIEW HOMEWORK AND OVERALL PROGRESS

As in earlier sessions, review last week's homework to provide an opportunity for reward and feedback. Discuss the child's reaction to the parents' chosen extinction task(s). For children who are having difficulty choosing and completing E/RP tasks toward the top of the symptom hierarchy, make it clear that continued effort is required and that it is not uncommon for things to slow down at this point in treatment. Be sure to compliment the child on progress to date. Communicate a sense of optimism about future gains.

## ADDRESS PLATEAUS

By this point in treatment, the child should have made significant gains and may even have reached a plateau. Plateaus (and there may be several during treatment) often indicate a need to consolidate the gains that have been made coupled with a need to "take a breather" before tackling more difficult E/RP tasks. Plateaus should be addressed by having ceremonies of graduation and by identifying the new "plane" or focus of treatment (i.e., by explicitly recognizing that the child has graduated to more difficult E/RP targets that are higher on the stimulus hierarchy). It is sometimes useful to redefine the transition/work zone by reapplying the cartographic metaphor used in Session 1 to demonstrate that OCD's circle is now considerably small, while the child's is much larger. The child is asked to consider what the new transition zone looks like and to choose a new aspect of OCD to attack. Note that the chosen target belongs to territory that was initially thought to be unreachable (i.e., involves symptoms that were initially rated a 10+ but are now 6–8 on the child's fear thermometer).

## CHOOSE HARDER E/RP TASKS

At this point, the therapist should encourage the child to consider an especially challenging exposure task for the coming week. While it is most important for the child to choose an exposure task that he or she is confident of completing, remind the child of past success with difficult tasks. It is sometimes possible to facilitate E/RP by appealing to the child's love of risk (e.g., by making analogies to roller coasters). When the child is embarking on very difficult E/RP tasks, the help of a cotherapist is often necessary. It can be quite helpful to engage a parent or friend to help with E/RP or schedule more frequent telephone check-ins with the therapist. On occasion, it may be necessary to schedule therapy sessions away from the office. Dialogue 13.1

illustrates how the therapist can help the child move past the plateau and tackle a more difficult level of E/RP tasks.

## Dialogue 13.1

MOM: Carla has made a good deal of progress, but she seems to have stopped trying over the past few weeks.

NADINE: You're right, Carla has done much to gain control over OCD and it does seem she has reached a plateau.

DAD: Does this mean she won't make any further progress?

NADINE: No, plateaus are not uncommon in treatment. It can, however, be helpful to do some special things to help Carla get over this plateau. One special intervention is to celebrate the gains Carla has already made so that she will feel she has gotten credit for them. Just as children need to have graduation ceremonies at school to encourage them toward the next higher and more difficult level, Carla needs to know that she too has graduated from an easy to a more difficult level of bossing back OCD. This will help her have the courage to regroup and begin in earnest on the next level.

MOM: But what if she doesn't want to go to the next level?

NADINE: That is possible, but only if the anxiety she must face seems too great. Part of treatment will include trying to break down the next level into more manageable pieces and helping Carla redefine her transition zone. If this is not possible, then I will work with Carla to choose a more difficult task this week that may require your help or the help of a friend.

NADINE: Carla, you have tackled a lot of Germy's territory and I think it's time to celebrate all that you have done so far.

CARLA: But Germy still bothers me when I'm at school and I don't think I can stop that.

NADINE: Yes, I know there is still some more territory to conquer, but you've graduated from the first level of bossing back OCD. Now you're entering the next level, which may be harder, but you can boss Germy back in the same way.

CARLA: How? it will be too hard!

NADINE: Remember when you touched the door knobs at home and your fear thermometer went up?

CARLA: Yes, but it came down pretty soon, and that doesn't bother me at all now.

NADINE: Exactly. Your fear thermometer will do the same thing when you tackle the bathroom doors at school—it will go up for a time, but then will come back down. How high do you think it might go?

CARLA: It would go up to an 8.

NADINE: Okay, do you think you can tolerate a level 8, now that you know it will come back down?

CARLA: I don't know, maybe if you or somebody was with me.

NADINE: Who would you like to go with you to touch the bathroom door at school?

CARLA: Well, my friend Susan could come. She knows about Germy and she tries to help me all the time.

NADINE: Okay, how about if you and Susan go to the bathroom door together after school and both of you touch it without washing your hands afterward?

CARLA: That would be hard, but I think I could do it with Susan there.

NADINE: Remember, you want to keep on touching the door until it gets to be boring. Okay?

CARLA: Okay, I'll try this week

## COMORBIDITY

As OCD subsides, comorbid conditions often move to center stage. Parents often feel frustrated when their child appears to acquire new problems. It is important to explain to parents that these problems were, in fact, always present, but were being masked or superseded by OCD. If further treatment and/or referral will eventually be necessary, the therapist should discuss this with the parents so that the focus on OCD is not watered down by preoccupation with other problems. However, comorbid conditions that are interfering with the treatment of OCD require prompt intervention so that the treatment of OCD itself does not become derailed. A not uncommon example of the former situation involves a shy child who has difficulty making friends. Parents may identify this as a problem and ask the therapist to intervene with the child to encourage friendships. A related issue emerges when the therapist identifies problems in the parents' marriage that do not have much to do with OCD but clearly cause distress to the parents. In both instances, the therapist may want to inquire about whether the newly identified source of suffering should become a focus of treatment once OCD is gone. If yes, then the structure of the new emphases in treatment should be mutually agreed upon (e.g., by including additional therapy sessions using a social phobia treatment protocol or referring the parents for marital therapy).

## PARENT CHECK-IN (SELECT PARENTS' E/RP TARGETS)

Parental extinction targets should usually continue to be chosen at the child's pace. Less commonly, when the child is unwilling or unable to give parents permission to stop participating in OCD rituals, parents are asked to select E/RP targets, even when the child protests. This strategy requires that the therapist (1) choose manageable E/RP targets (especially when parents desire too rapid an improvement) and (2) provide parents with a strategy for managing the child's distress. In some cases, when family members are extensively involved in rituals, they will need to play a more central role in treatment. Dialogue 13.2 illustrates how the therapist can work with parents and child to select extinction targets and learn how to manage resulting anxiety.

### Dialogue 13.2

NADINE: Carla has told me she insists that you tell her how you checked all the door and window locks before bed.

MOM: Yes, each night we have to go through the same ritual and, if I miss a door or window, I have to start over.

CARLA: I've decided you don't have to do that anymore.

NADINE: Carla and I also talked about how this will make her anxiety go up and she may have a hard time not asking you over and over anyway.

MOM: What do we do then?

NADINE: You will need a strategy for helping Carla with her anxiety, such as a cue for her to use her relaxation exercises or do a fun activity. Carla, what would you like your parents to say if you start getting anxious and ask them extra questions?

CARLA: I don't know—they could not answer, but then I'd probably get madder.

NADINE: How would it be if they remind you Germy is in the room and take a deep breath as a cue for you to begin to relax?

CARLA: That might be okay.

NADINE: Another strategy would be to do something else to help your mind get off Germy. Does anyone have an idea for a fun activity to do before bed?

DAD: Sometime we read aloud before bed. We could always have a good book to be reading together.

CARLA: Yeah, that would be good. We could read a chapter book.

NADINE: Okay, so when Germy gives you extra anxiety because your parents aren't telling you about the locks, your parents will cue you with a deep breath and then will get the chapter book. Is that okay?

CARLA AND PARENTS: Yes, that's worth a try.


## EVALUATION

The therapist should spend a few minutes charting ratings on the NIMH Global OC Scale and on the CGI scales. The therapist should also obtain ratings on the YBOCS during treatment weeks 12 and 16 (usually Sessions 14 and 18).


## HOMEWORK

• Homework should be to practice an E/RP task or tasks taken from the revised stimulus hierarchy discussed during this session.

• Remind the parents and the child that, in the middle of treatment, patients typically will have internalized the strategy and be able to apply it to targets that were not specifically identified as homework. (Within the framework of a single case design, this if often called generalizing across the baselines.) While in general this is a good thing, tackling E/RP targets that were not first rehearsed in therapy can result in the child being overmatched, with the end result that OCD is strengthened. In contrast to the rapid progress in the middle of therapy, things often slow down a bit when the child hits the upper end of the stimulus hierarchy since these are the most difficult E/RP targets to tackle and produce the most anxiety. It is important to reassure the child who is now approaching these more difficult tasks that selecting one target per week and completely habituating to that target is a worthy goal and not a failure after the relatively easy successes of earlier weeks.

• If the exposure task is particularly difficult, the child may choose to enlist the help of a family member or friend as a cotherapist.

The therapist should schedule a midweek telephone call to encourage the child in the E/RP task and assess the need to modify the E/RP program.

# Chapter 14

## Session 19: Relapse Prevention

Carla feels like OCD is gone; Germy has been squashed! She knows, however, that OCD can surprise her again at any time. Nadine asks her to think about how Germy might try to make a "come back." Carla says it would probably be with bathroom worries. During this week's session and over the following week, Carla does some extra E/RP tasks involving several different public bathrooms. Her anxiety does not rise very high while doing these exposure tasks, but she knows this practice will help her if Germy tries to regain lost territory in the future.

### GOALS OF SESSION 19

1. Explain concept of relapse prevention.
2. Provide opportunity for imaginal exposure.
3. Address questions or concerns regarding the end of treatment.

### REVIEW HOMEWORK

As always, review the past week's homework to provide an opportunity for reward and feedback. For children who are having difficulty with the final E/RP tasks, make it clear that continued effort is required. Be sure to compliment the child on progress to date. Communicate a sense of optimism about future gains, even though residual symptoms remain as treatment nears its end.

## EXPLAIN RELAPSE PREVENTION

Now that OCD symptoms are much reduced, it is necessary to introduce the concept of relapse prevention. The child may prefer not to think of the possibility of relapse; however, addressing relapse is in itself a necessary exposure task in the child's struggle against OCD. We frequently use the terms "slip" or "lapse" to refer to brief and expectable symptom flare-ups, which we distinguish from a "relapse" in which OCD makes a substantial and persistent return appearance despite the child's best efforts to resist. In this way, we help the child realize that "slips" don't mean the loss of all that has been gained throughout CBT treatment. Slips are not a failure, but something that happens with OCD. Fortunately, slips are time limited and, with appropriate intervention, are easily relieved (i.e., it is generally possible to prevent slips from turning into a relapse by using the strategies the child has learned in treatment).

## FACILITATE IMAGINAL EXPOSURE

It has been postulated that the durability of the improvement seen with CBT as contrasted with medication is due to the internalization of the CBT techniques. The goal of this session is, therefore, to reinforce such internalization so that the child will automatically do the opposite of what OCD asks. In relapse prevention, the child is asked to imagine an expectable "slip," which he or she successfully fights back by using the "tool kit." Ask the child to describe the symptom OCD would most likely use to try to reclaim territory. Encourage the child to imagine the slip as if it were really happening and to be specific and detailed in order to facilitate imaginal exposure. During exposure, the child rates his or her anxiety at 1- to 2-minute intervals using the fear thermometer. As anxiety peaks, remind the child to use the tool kit, especially constructive self-talk. When the child's fear level has returned to zero, the exposure task is complete.

After completing this task, run through all the major classes of symptoms enumerated on the YBOCS Symptom Checklist. Discuss with the child how each major subtype of OCD might appear, and initiate a brief imaginal exposure task to rehearse applying the tool kit to prevent OCD from establishing itself. Dialogue 19.1 illustrates a graduation exercise in understanding relapse prevention.

*Dialogue 19.1*

NADINE: Carla, let's say that OCD tries to make a comeback 2 or 3 years from now. Imagine that you are walking down the hall at school when you suddenly get the paralyzing fear that if you touch the door knob and then touch your mouth, you'll get AIDS and infect your whole family so that you will all die a terrible death. What would you do?

CARLA: Well, first I'd say, "Hello, OCD," because I'd recognize that thought as typical OCD stuff. Then I'd tell OCD that I really didn't have time to play, and I'd grab the door knob, touch my mouth, and go off to the library using the tools I learned here to calm myself down as best I could.

NADINE: Whoopee, you get an A+!

If the child has been receiving medication for OCD, it is important for the therapist to emphasize that it is the child who has been responsible for eliminating or reducing OCD symptoms, and that the medication was merely a help (e.g., as water wings are in learning to swim). Otherwise, the child may attribute success to the medication, which increases the possibility of relapse when medication is withdrawn. The therapist should remind parents and child that booster CBT sessions will be needed when the child eventually stops medication in order to reduce the risk of relapse.

## WHAT HAPPENS AFTER TREATMENT?

The fear caused by a slip is related not only to the OCD symptom itself, but also to concern about the loss of treatment gains (e.g., a total relapse). While acknowledging that OCD is sometimes a recurring problem, the therapist should reinforce the idea that relapse is unlikely, since the child now has a set of strategies and allies plus lots of experience combating OCD.

Adolescents, in particular, often ask questions about the chronicity of OCD. As part of relapse prevention, the therapist and child should discuss how OCD affects development. While it is not possible to anticipate all the possible issues that might arise in such a conversation, existential issues often come up during these end-of-treatment sessions. For example, the young person may wonder about the impact of OCD on future happiness (e.g., "Can I pass it onto my kids?") or about how to fill the new space freed up as OCD remits (e.g., "How do I ask a girl out?"). Addressing such issues early in treatment frequently constitutes an avoidance behavior; however, failure to address them now may inhibit the normal transition out of OCD treatment.

Depending on the child's temperament and the family history of mental illness, the therapist may wish to briefly review the developmentally based risk for other mental illnesses (e.g., teenage depression or social phobia).

Finally, we never "terminate" treatment, but rather leave the door open in case patients need to return to work on OCD or other psychiatric problems.

## PARENT CHECK-IN

While parents should be encouraged to praise the child for resisting OCD slips, the main emphasis for the parent should now be on relapse prevention and focusing attention on positive elements in the child's life. The therapist should be sure that parents understand the potential for relapse and slips, so that they can help their child address these slips as soon as they occur. Parents should be encouraged to maintain an alert but matter-of-fact attitude about the possibility of relapse and not to be surprised by such an "attack."

The therapist should also inform parents of the necessity for booster CBT sessions in the future, should OCD try to make a "come back." It is helpful to be frank with parents of children with severe OCD about the reality of persistent symptoms and the likelihood of symptom exacerbation in the future. Parents should be encouraged, however, by the fact that they and their child have learned strategies and tools to fight OCD that can be used at any time, with any "flavor" of OCD.

During this session, the therapist should also discuss plans for upcoming graduation ceremonies with parents.

## EVALUATION

The therapist should spend a few minutes charting ratings on the NIMH Global OC Scale and on the CGI scales.

## HOMEWORK

- This week's homework task consists of a relapse prevention exposure task done imaginally or in vivo.
- The child may also wish to choose another exposure task on the symptom hierarchy that has not yet been satisfactorily accomplished even if the symptom is subclinical.
- As with all exposure tasks, the fear thermometer is used to rate anxiety until it attenuates.

# Chapter 15

# Session 20: Graduation

Carla is excited because today is her "graduation day." Nadine presents Carla with a certificate of accomplishment and they discuss how Carla will celebrate her achievement. Carla and her parents are full of stories of bossing Germy back. Yesterday during Art, Carla got paint on her hands and was unable to wash it all off, but went on to eat lunch anyway. "Germy didn't bother me at all—he's off my land for good." Carla is now able to do many things that OCD used to prevent. Over the weekend, Carla went to a friend's house to spend the night and Germy was nowhere to be found, not even in the bathroom sink.

## GOALS OF SESSION 20

1. Celebrate the child's accomplishments.
2. Present the child with a certificate of achievement.
3. Encourage the child to notify friends and/or family members about his or her success.

## CELEBRATE THE CHILD'S ACCOMPLISHMENTS

This session focuses on the accomplishments the child has made throughout the treatment process. In other words, it is a "brag" session, during which the child is encouraged to recognize the specific territory he or she has reclaimed from OCD. Recalling the process helps to cement the child's new story or map, a map without OCD. Although the possibility that OCD will try to reclaim territory is directly acknowledged, emphasis is placed on the ability the child has acquired to "boss back" OCD. The child's new story is made even more concrete by presenting a certificate of achievement.

## PRESENT CERTIFICATE OF ACHIEVEMENT

We present a certificate of achievement to the child on which the therapist has penned congratulations for a job well done. Much like the Tin Man's heart, the Lion's badge, or the Scarecrow's diploma in the *Wizard of Oz*, the certificate of achievement is a tangible reminder of the skills that the child can now draw upon when confronting OCD. The child no longer needs to hide from OCD, but can proudly notify others that OCD is under his or her control.

## ENCOURAGE NOTIFICATION

Notifying family and friends solidifies the gains made against OCD. The child's triumph over OCD is a testament to his or her competence and contrasts sharply with former dysfunction or failure. Many children may still be reluctant to tell others about OCD and often prefer to keep the treatment process a secret. While it is not necessary to tell everyone, the therapist should encourage the child to tell at least one peer or valued adult of his or her accomplishments.

## PARENT CHECK-IN

During this session, it is important that the therapist address any lingering concerns parents may have and discuss follow-up issues. Parents should be reminded of the CBT booster session scheduled in 6 weeks and of the availability of future booster sessions, should OCD try to make a "come back." For many children, monthly or bimonthly sessions will be necessary to manage residual OCD symptoms.

## EVALUATION

The therapist should obtain ratings on the YBOCS, the NIMH Global OC Scale, and the CGI scales during Session 20. For many children and parents, reviewing the downward course of OCD symptoms over time provides a nice visual confirmation of how far they have all come in "bossing back OCD."

## HOMEWORK

- The child's homework is to notify the family members and friends chosen during the session about his or her success over OCD. This can be done verbally or by showing off the certificate of achievement.
- One final homework task might be to frame or display the child's certificate.
- An appointment is made for a 6-week booster session.

# Chapter 16

## Session 21: Booster Session

Carla reports that "Germy is nowhere to be seen." Mostly, she wants to talk about all the new and exciting things that she's doing with her friends. With careful questioning, she reports using her CBT strategies when Germy tried to make her afraid of eating in a restaurant. Another time she sought out the dog to pet after Germy planted a series of thoughts in her mind about the dog making her sick with rabies. Otherwise, Carla has had no OCD symptoms at all. After describing these episodes, Carla comments, "You're a good coach. I've got it, don't I?" To which Nadine replies, "Yes, Carla, you've got it."

### GOALS OF SESSION 21

1. Celebrate the child's accomplishments.
2. Review the toolkit.
3. Reinforce relapse prevention.
4. Plan notifications regarding the end of treatment.

### CHECK-IN

The focus of this session is to solidify the child's sense of accomplishment, with particular attention to making sure that the child attributes success to him- or herself rather than to the therapist or to medication.

153

The therapist begins the session by reviewing the past 6 weeks for residual and new OCD symptoms, focusing on how the child has used his or her CBT strategies to (hopefully) successfully manage any new or residual OCD symptoms.

## REVIEW THE TOOL KIT

Having established the current state of OCD, the therapist then reviews each tool in the child's tool kit. The therapist and child should recall an example of how the child used each tool to beat OCD during the treatment phase, and if needed, during the period between the end of treatment and today's booster session. Finally, in order to reinforce relapse prevention and generalization training, the therapist should repeat the most pertinent imaginal exposure exercises learned during Session 19.

## PARENT CHECK-IN

As always, parents are encouraged to provide feedback concerning their child's progress. Since this is the last scheduled session, it is important that the therapist address any lingering concerns or questions about follow-up that parents may have. In particular, parents should be informed that they can reach you at any time if the child is having difficulty with OCD and needs additional booster sessions. Also, if the child has been receiving medication, parents should be asked to schedule several booster sessions during the period when medication withdrawal will be attempted. It is our practice to decrease medication by 25% every 2–3 months after the child has been in stable remission for 6–12 months, and to schedule two booster sessions at the time of each successive drop in medications.

## EVALUATION

As appropriate, the therapist may wish to obtain final ratings on the YBOCS, the NIMH Global OC Scale, and the CGI scales during the Booster Session.

## HOMEWORK

• Today's homework is for the child to notify family members and friends that treatment is completed.

• Follow-up visits may be scheduled from every month to every 3 months, depending on how solidly the child has banished OCD and on developmental transitions and life events that my be upcoming. In general, visits at intervals of 3 months make sense during the first year, after which we see children yearly just to "check in."

# Part Three

# TROUBLESHOOTING

The best way to learn is to go out and makes mistakes as
fast as possible.

—*Jim Gustafson, MD*

Though most children benefit from treatment as outlined in Part II of
this manual, not all benefit equally and an unfortunate few show little,
if any, response. For example, some children have OCD symptoms that
are not as readily amenable to E/RP, while others don't tolerate E/RP
well because of somatic/automonic symptoms or motor restlessness.
This section focuses on identifying and overcoming pitfalls that commonly complicate the treatment of OCD so that you, the therapist,
can get treatment moving in the right direction even when OCD is
at its most difficult. In Chapter 17, we describe common pitfalls that
can interfere with successful treatment. Chapter 18 addresses treatment components that can be added to standard care to successfully
manage variations in symptom presentation. Families and schools
often get tangled up with OCD; thus, it is important for therapists to
help disentangle family members and school personnel from OCD. In
Chapters 19 and 20, we discuss how to tackle problems at home and
at school. Using the approaches presented in these last three chapters,
the therapist can identify and manage most common pitfalls in the
implementation of CBT so that treatment can move forward again.

# Chapter 17

## Pitfalls

In a 1995 review of the literature on CBT for pediatric OCD, one of us (JSM) wrote, "Abundant clinical evidence suggests that cognitive-behavioral psychotherapy, alone or in combination with pharmacotherapy, is an effective treatment for OCD in children and adolescents. . . . Helping patients make rapid and difficult behavior change over short time intervals takes considerable skill" (March, 1995). While these words continue to ring true—CBT is still the only effective psychotherapeutic intervention for pediatric OCD (March & Mulle, 1996)—not everybody benefits and not all children benefit equally. Thus, considerable room for treatment innovation remains. In this regard, a large part of what differentiates a competent from an expert cognitive-behavioral psychotherapist is the ability to understand and successfully address so-called "pitfalls" in treatment. Table 17.1 lists some common reasons why CBT may yield insufficient benefit, which we discuss in this chapter. Those interested in a more in-depth discussion will find that a close reading of the book *Failures in Behavioral Therapy* by Foa and Emmelkamp (1983) is also well worth the effort.

**TABLE 17.1.** Reasons for Treatment Failure

Inexpert CBT
Lack of compassion
Developmental factors
Symptomatic pitfalls in implementing CBT
Need for medication: differentiating CBT and medication
Comorbidity

## THERAPIST FACTORS

Inexpert CBT

Perhaps the most common reason CBT fails to show benefit is inexpert CBT. Many patients referred to our clinic as treatment resistant have not actually received CBT! For example, it is not uncommon for patients to describe having had relaxation or biofeedback training. Since relaxation is often used as an active placebo in OCD treatment studies (Marks, 1987), it isn't surprising that these patients did not do well. On average, 12 to 20 sessions of therapist-assisted, hierarchy-based E/RP is the average necessary course of CBT, without which most patients are unlikely to get better.

Even when therapists use hierarchy-based E/RP, most children and adolescents don't do well if therapists essentially tell them just to stop doing OCD rituals. Most children would already have done so if they could. What is missing in such situations is a structured and developmentally sensitive approach to CBT. For example, using the transition zone to allow the child to choose E/RP targets in a predictable and controllable fashion goes a long way toward solving the central problem of how to select E/RP targets. The wise therapist will read widely in the OCD literature, paying close attention to the clinical pearls inherent in our approach, while adapting CBT to his or her own unique clinical style.

Lack of Compassion

As mental health professionals, we haven't been very good over the years at making the problem—in this case OCD—the problem. Rather, we have typically used a panoply of terms—resistance, denial, and sabotage are among the more common—with which to blame patients and their families for the fact that treatment isn't going well. Parents often fall into the same trap, assuming that lack of motivation accounts for their child's slow progress. Not surprisingly, then, the child with OCD often feels that other people lack compassion for the difficulties inherent in E/RP, which is why making OCD the problem is a cornerstone of the treatment approach outlined in this book.

When therapy stalls, it is not uncommon for therapists (and parents) to have the urge to tighten the screws on the child, assuming that he or she isn't trying hard enough. This may be the correct approach to disruptive behaviors that are not related to OCD. For example, while OCD may interfere with children's ability to do certain household chores, some children inappropriately use OCD as an excuse to avoid chores that do not involve OCD triggers. Such a youngster may be more motivated to work on OCD if other aspects of family life are adjusted to take into account what is (and is not) related to OCD. Nonetheless, when therapy for OCD stalls, it is usually because the child is stuck on a particular E/RP target or set of targets. In this case, simply suggesting that the child may have aimed too high on the hierarchy, or even that it is time for "a week off," will begin to move treatment forward again. In this sense, the job of the therapist as coach is to counsel patience, allowing the negative reinforcement value of OCD to get the therapeutic process moving again. Consequently, we *never* use terms such as resistance or sabotage, preferring instead to ask if we might be missing something, such as a complicating comorbid condition, before concluding that OCD is sufficiently severe that our best efforts and those of the patient are simply insufficient.

## Where Therapists Fear to Tread

Some children and adolescents present with OCD symptoms that may pose moral or personal challenges to some if not all therapists. Two examples illustrate the point. In the first, a young man presents with the obsession that looking at another man's body signals a homosexual advance. Despite a complete lack of any homosexual leanings or experiences, this teenager is unable to tolerate being in another room with men, including his father, and cannot read any material that includes content regarding homosexuality. A skilled therapist would help gradually expose this young man to increasingly difficult-to-tolerate materials and settings that challenge the obsession and accompanying avoidance behaviors. But what if the therapist believes that homosexuality is "sinful" and is personally so uncomfortable that the necessary exposure to homosexual content becomes too difficult for the therapist? Even worse, what if the patient shares these beliefs so that the patient and therapist are both conflicted about the issue? In a second example, a patient is phobic about contamination with germs, especially germs on toilet seats. In E/RP she must touch a public toilet seat and refrain from washing. But what if the therapist cannot easily model and thus structure such an E/RP task because of his own fastidiousness? Clearly, the therapist cannot lead the patient in a direction that she cannot go herself, which makes the ability to take risks and to tolerate uncertainty critical for therapists who work with OCD patients. While cognitive therapy approaches may be used to challenge restricting beliefs—for example, beliefs about the need for cleanliness that are clearly unskillful—E/RP is not about meaning, which to some extent must be suspended in order to habituate OCD symptoms. Hence, when uncomfortable with some element of OCD, the therapist must confront his or her own uneasiness with the content of the obsession so that E/RP can move forward, since "going beyond normal" is one key to recovery from OCD. Once the patient has accomplished the necessary E/RP task, then "what's appropriate or normal" is up to the patient and family to decide. When the therapist cannot model the necessary E/RP tasks, securing supervision with a more experienced cognitive-behavioral psychotherapist may help the therapist overcome his or her own limitations. For others, it may be better to leave certain classes of OCD patients to someone else if the content of the obsessions is too troubling to be managed.

## DEVELOPMENTAL FACTORS

In our experience, the cognitive-behavioral strategies used in this treatment protocol are reliably effective in children as young as 5 and as old as 18. Nonetheless, as we point out in discussing developmental considerations for each treatment session, CBT procedures should be adjusted to each patient's level of cognitive functioning, social maturity, and capacity for sustained attention. The therapist should keep developmental considerations in mind and be flexible in structuring the treatments within the constraints of the fixed session goals. Cognitive interventions, especially, require adjustment to the developmental level of the patient. For example, adolescents are typically less likely to appreciate giving OCD a nasty nickname than younger children. A few children with exceptionally concrete thinking styles may wish to externalize OCD as an unfortunate habit for which they can assume responsibility. Patients whose OCD symptoms entangle family members will require more family involvement in treatment planning and implementation than those without family involvement. Nevertheless, while developmental considerations should be kept in mind throughout the treatment, the general format and goals of the treatment sessions will be the same for all children.

## SYMPTOMATIC PITFALLS IN IMPLEMENTING CBT

Table 17.2 lists some common symptomatic pitfalls that can interfere with the implementation of CBT.

**TABLE 17.2.** Common Symptomatic
Pitfalls in Implementing CBT

Mental rituals
Reassurance seeking
"Bailing out"
Hasty rituals
Delayed rituals
Performance anxiety
Myth of cure
Excessive focus on medication
Constraints within the family (see Chapter
19 for a discussion of these issues)

## Mental Rituals

When a child fails to habituate despite adequate duration of exposure, he or she may be using mental rituals to decrease anxiety within the E/RP task, in effect replacing the previous compulsion. Some common mental rituals include: turning OCD on its head by saying, "If I do the ritual, something bad will happen;" silently noting that it will be sufficient to perform the ritual (e.g., washing) the next possible time; inventing a whole new ritual (e.g., praying); subtly reassuring oneself *in loco parentis* by recalling previous instances of reassurance; or simply saying, "It doesn't matter this time." Once identified, these mental rituals can be placed on the hierarchy and eliminated. Be aware, however, that the use of mental rituals may indicate that the chosen E/RP task is actually too hard and that it would be appropriate to back down the hierarchy somewhat.

## Reassurance Seeking

Children are very good at seeking reassurance from adults or peers— and doing so is a useful social skill in many circumstances. However, if the child engages in reassurance seeking as an escape–avoidance behavior, then an extinction procedure is necessary. It is important to be aware that reassurance seeking can be overt or covert and verbal or nonverbal. Examples of overt reassurance seeking include asking a direct question or looking for sympathetic reassurance in a facial expression. Snuggling or inappropriate clinging to escape anxiety or delay exposure are examples of covert but still obvious nonverbal reassurance seeking. Covert verbal reassurance seeking can be quite subtle. For example, a child may ask about a future event unrelated to an E/RP task to reassure himself that future consequences have been averted. Once identified, these escape–avoidance behaviors must be blocked in order for habituation to occur.

### "Bailing Out"

Anxiety may also remain unchanged after several practice exposures if the child has not waited during the exposure task for his or her "temperature" on the fear thermometer to come down to a level of 2 or below. Although dysphoric affects generally decrease within 20 or 30 minutes, it is not unusual for anxiety to take up to an hour or more to reach baseline. Using the fear thermometer to construct habituation curves by rating anxiety at intervals throughout the exposure task is one way for the child to ensure he or she does not discontinue the exposure task prematurely (i.e., before anxiety habituates). When escape–avoidance within E/RP is a frequent problem, however, the usual solution is to back down the stimulus hierarchy to guarantee success. Even rare escape–avoidance is a big problem, since caving in and doing a ritual after initially trying to resist exerts a strong reinforcing effect on the side of OCD. Under these circumstances, it is better to suggest to the child that he think of E/RP as a "Y" or fork in the road. Once the child has headed down the E/RP side of the "Y," he or she has to stick it out. If starting E/RP seems too hard, however, there is no shame in taking the other branch, namely avoiding contrived exposure entirely or, with uncontrived exposure, resisting the ritual as much as possible. It is usually better to acknowledge that OCD is stronger "this time" than to try and fail.

### "Hasty Rituals"

Many children try to get their homework or their chores done as fast as possible so that they can go outside and play or watch television. It is no different with OCD—children often use a "hasty rituals" strategy to get rituals done as quickly and with as little interference as possible. This approach, of course, blocks any chance of habituation. Fortunately, E/RP homework generally takes little more, and some-times takes less, time than the hastily performed ritual. Since the goal is always to go play, pointing this out to the child sometimes has a very beneficial effect on moving E/RP along. Note also that hastily done rituals most often fall within the transition zone and thus make excellent candidates for properly done E/RP. Finally, if the E/RP task involves limiting the time taken to do a ritual that requires a certain number of repetitions, make sure that the child isn't using the "hasty rituals" strategy to cram all the repetitions into a shorter time span.

## Delayed Rituals

In some cases, children seem to have habituated across successive E/RP trials, but the identified triggers for OCD do not disappear from the hierarchy because the child is *actually* doing the ritual on a delayed basis. For example, a child may delay praying, washing, or checking until no one else is around. The only way to know about delayed rituals—unless a parent discovers the child ritualizing without an obvious trigger—is to ask. If the child is delaying rituals, then response prevention is the treatment of choice. If the child needs help, it may be necessary to set up support structures to help the child succeed in stopping delayed rituals. For example, the youngster who is washing late at night when everyone else has gone to bed may need permission to sleep in the same room with a sibling or parent for a week or two while he habituates to that particular E/RP task.

## Performance Anxiety

When a therapist, parent, or teacher is impatiently waiting for a child to show improvement, the child may resist E/RP because of fear of failure, fear of disappointing others, or feeling pressured. Fear of failure leads to excessive self-criticism; fear of disappointing others, or even worse, doing so, makes the child become reluctant to risk failure; and feeling pressured leads to an "on strike" reaction with the child feeling that no improvement will ever be good enough. Performance anxiety is especially common in children with social phobia and/or when the child is frequently praised for no reason except to prop up his or her self-esteem. The natural tendency of parents to want to help children feel better generally backfires. Helping parents minimize noncontingent reinforcement allows the child to undertake E/RP without worrying about disappointing family members. Parents generally understand this approach if the therapist simply points out that defeating OCD will do more for self-esteem than all the praise in the world. The pent-up demand for the child to stop inconveniencing other people with OCD is more problematic. When everyone wants OCD over and done with, the child may worry (often correctly) that a micron of improvement will dramatically increase demands that he or she simply stop doing rituals. This is especially common when OCD has caused a formerly good student to fail or when parents are missing work or fighting between themselves over OCD. In this case, you can control the structure of the treatment by counseling parents to be patient, just as you would do with the parents of a child with any other medical illness. Using the stimulus hierarchy to define the transition/work zone to parents as the only place where E/RP is possible is the key to increasing the child's willingness to tackle E/RP tasks. As discussed in Chapter 20, it is also important to help school personnel make appropriate accommodations for a sick child, since OCD may compromise much of the school year depending on the child's response to treatment.

## Myth of Cure

Naturally, everyone wants OCD to disappear, and the culture of psychotherapy since Freud has believed cure not only possible, but expectable, given good therapy. Fortunately, most patients make considerable improvement with CBT alone or CBT plus medications. Unfortunately, only 20–30% of our patients go into complete remission; another 5–10% remain quite ill despite good treatment. Most patients still have some OCD symptoms with which to contend even at the successful conclusion of treatment. For this reason, it is important to point out to the child and parents from the beginning of therapy that OCD is a lifelong medical illness that likely will wax and wane. This helps all concerned adjust to the likely outcome of treatment—namely, that the child will be very much to much improved but is likely to continue to have residual symptoms. In this regard, we tell our patients that the goal of therapy is subclinical OCD—that is, nobody knows that the OCD is still hanging around a little but the child, who feels comfortable keeping OCD at bay.

## Excessive Focus on Medication

Pills are powerful aids, and the mythology associated with them can unfortunately invite patients and their parents to do nothing while they wait for the medication to magically make OCD go away. There are three reasons why this attitude is counterproductive. First, the benefits of medication fortuitously achieve their maximum effect between treatment weeks 8–12, just when the patient is reaching the top of the stimulus hierarchy, so that a good case can be made for combining medication with CBT, especially in the very ill patient. Moreover, empirical literature tells us that treatment with a serotonin reuptake inhibitor typically results in a 30–40% decrease in OCD symptoms, which translates into reports of moderate to marked improvement when patients are asked how well they are doing compared to before starting treatment. However, fewer than 20% of patients treated with medication alone in clinical studies reach subclinical status, suggesting that medication is helpful but not a panacea for most patients (March, Leonard, & Swedo, 1995; March, Frances, et al., 1997).

Second, the great majority of patients relapse when medications are withdrawn unless the patient has received concomitant CBT, which adds durability to treatment results (Leonard, Lenane, et al., 1991).

Third, a study by Marks and colleagues convincingly demonstrated that antiexposure instructions completely attenuate the benefits of medication. In this study, patients treated with clomipramine and E/RP did very well. Another group were instructed to avoid the things that triggered OCD, and when avoidance wasn't possible, to do their rituals willingly. The antiexposure instructions eliminated any medication effect in this group, so that E/RP seems to be necessary for medication to work rather than the other way around! We almost always describe this study when pointing out to parents why it is better to make CBT explicit, as in this program, rather than to rely on implicit, haphazard resistance to OCD (Marks et al., 1988).

Whatever the combination of symptoms and patient preferences that influence the choice to start a medication, we typically refer to medication as "water wings" to convey the notion that it is the child's efforts in CBT, just like his or her efforts at swimming, that provide the payoff. Using this approach, and emphasizing the therapy process variables outlined in this handbook, we have almost no CBT refusers, and the tendency to rely on medications rather than doing the hard work of E/RP is minimized.


## NEED FOR MEDICATION: DIFFERENTIATING CBT AND MEDICATION

As noted earlier, most children present to mental health settings because of problematic behaviors either in relationships or in the school setting. The clinician's task is to understand these behaviors in the context of the constraints to normal development that underlie them. While many behaviors are in some sense problematic, not all behaviors, even symptomatic behaviors, are appropriate targets for medication management or, for that matter, for CBT. For example, in the child with ADHD, standing patiently in line is an appropriate target for contingency management whereas decreased sensation-seeking and increased vigilance may be more appropriate targets for medication management. It is crucial to clearly define the target symptoms for psychopharmacological as contrasted to psychosocial interventions wherever possible. With OCD, we usually use the analogy of a dimmer switch for a light bulb to communicate the idea that pharmacotherapy decreases obsessions and their accompanying affects, while at the same time making it easier to resist OCD. Conversely, only the child can make the choice to resist OCD, which is why a structured CBT program built around making skillful choices is so helpful for most young persons with the disorder.

Like many experts (March, Frances, et al., 1997), we usually recommend starting with CBT alone when possible. However, patients with severe OCD or with complicating conditions, such as panic disorder or depression that may interfere with CBT, will frequently wish to start with medication, adding CBT once the medicine has provided some symptomatic relief. If a patient has started with weekly CBT alone, and satisfactory progress has not been made within 6–10 weeks despite a strong effort by the patient to resist OCD, adding medications is usually a good idea. For many patients, starting both treatments from the beginning will be attractive because combined treatment offers the possibility of greater benefit, especially for the most difficult-to-resist OCD symptoms. Although we see many patients who have "failed" multiple medication trials, it is our experience that returning to standard well-delivered pharmacotherapy plus CBT plus an academic intervention if needed converts nonresponders to responders more reliably than polypharmacy.

## COMORBIDITY

As mentioned in the introductory chapters of this manual, comorbid conditions can complicate both the diagnosis and treatment of pediatric OCD. In some cases, the presence of a comorbid disorder, such as a tic or thought disorder, indicates the need for an additional treatment, such as a neuroleptic medication, that is both augmentative (for the OCD) and adjunctive (for the comorbidity). In other cases, the treatments, such as stimulants for ADHD, target different symptom constellations (March, Wells, & Conners, 1995; March, Wells, &

Conners, 1996). In a comprehensive discussion of the influence of comorbidity on treatment planning, Clarkin and Kendall make the obvious but often neglected point that treatments must be matched to their targets (Clarkin & Kendall, 1992). We generally recommend parsimoniously combining treatments that are appropriate for OCD and/or for the comorbid conditions, while carefully monitoring treatment outcomes for each intervention (March, Leonard, et al., 1995; March, Frances, et al., 1997). For example, disruptive behavior disorders (DRBs) can be conceptualized in part as problems of reward salience; thus, the treatments for DRBs manipulate rewards and punishments, while using cognitive training to help the patient cope with anger (March, Wells, & Conners, 1996). Depression can be conceptualized as a problem of loss in relationships. In CBT for depression, the therapist works to help the patient change thoughts and behaviors in a way that leads to better relationships, whether intrapsychic, interpersonal, work, or spiritual. In anxiety disorders, CBT targets cognitions and behaviors designed to promote habituation or extinction of inappropriate fears, as we have seen in this program for the treatment of pediatric OCD with CBT. Each of these treatments is supported by a robust research literature, and manuals are available to guide practitioners in using CBT for specific problems.

Table 17.3 lists some common treatment combinations and provides pointers to the appropriate CBT literature (full citations are provided in the reference section). When CBT is listed, it is assumed that interventions for OCD will be blended with those for the other disorders as appropriate.

## MULTIMODAL "TEAM" TREATMENT

It should be clear by now that successful treatment of pediatric OCD requires the clinician to play a variety of professional roles, including supportive psychotherapist, behavior therapist, psychopharmacologist, and perhaps, family therapist. Few mental health providers are equally skilled in all these areas (e.g., psychiatrists are often poorly trained in behavioral treatments and psychologists in medication). Furthermore, in many settings such as large multispecialty groups or community mental health centers, child psychiatrists regularly function as diagnostic and psychopharmacologic consultants, with other aspects of OCD treatment provided by professionals from other disciplines. Especially in such settings, initiation of a multimodal treatment plan for a child with OCD requires a team approach in which different providers carry out

**TABLE 17.3.** Treatment Recommendations for OCD Complicated
by Comorbid Conditions

| Comorbid disorder | First-line treatment | Reference to CBT literature |
|---|---|---|
| OC spectrum disorder | SRI + CBT | Peterson, Campise, & Azrin (1994) |
| Tourette syndrome | CBT + SRI + neuroleptic | Peterson et al. (1994) |
| Panic disorder or social phobia | CBT + SRI or CBT alone | Barlow & Craske (1989) |
| Depression | CBT + SRI | Lewinsohn, Clarke, & Rohde (1994) |
| Bipolar I or II (in remission on mood stabilizer alone) | CBT + mood stabilizer ± SRI | Lewinsohn, Clarke, & Rohnde (1994) |
| Schizophrenia | SRI + neuroleptic | McEvoy et al. (1996) |
| Attention-deficit/ hyperactivity disorder | CBT + SRI + psychostimulant | Barkley (1995) |
| Disruptive behaviors | SRI + CBT + family therapy | Barkley (1995) |

*Note.* SRI = serotonin reuptake inhibitor; CBT = cognitive-behavioral therapy.

different aspects of the treatment program in a coordinated fashion.
With each individual on the team coming from a potentially different
theoretical orientation, each person's role must be subsumed under a
common neurobehavioral framework such as the one outlined in this
manual. Such an approach may enable many children previously labeled
as treatment-resistant to become treatment responders. Consideration
should be given to referring those children who do not respond readily
to standard treatments or who have complex medical or psychiatric
conditions to an OCD subspecialty clinic for consultation or definitive
treatment.

## FAMILY AND SCHOOL CONSTRAINTS

As noted throughout this book, family and school issues come up
repeatedly in the care of children with OCD. OCD may tangle up
family members and/or interfere with school, or problems at home

and/or at school may constrain the implementation of treatment for OCD. Because disentangling family members and school personnel from OCD is one key to successful treatment, we cover OCD at home and in the school setting in detail in Chapters 19 and 20, respectively.

## SUMMARY

Many so-called "difficult-to-manage" children with OCD have not had the benefit of skillful treatment. Ideally, all children with OCD should receive CBT optimized for children and adolescents. If they do not rapidly respond to CBT, a serotonin reuptake inhibitor should be added. For children with more severe OCD and those with complicating comorbid conditions, it may be appropriate to begin with medication treatment, since CBT may not be possible without medication support. Some children and families in this situation may prefer to try CBT alone, in hopes of avoiding the need for medication and accompanying side effects. Although current treatments are not curative, given a correct diagnosis and skillful treatment, most children can be helped to resume a normal developmental trajectory.

Chapter 18

# Special Wrinkles: Supplemental Treatment Interventions

As Lee Baer points out in *Getting Control* (Baer, 1991), many OCD patients exhibit symptoms that do not fall neatly within the scope of standard treatment interventions. Perhaps E/RP is difficult because of high levels of muscle tension and restlessness. Panic-level anxiety, including difficulty breathing, may interfere with E/RP. The patient's OCD may involve primarily mental phenomena and rituals that are not easily accessible to E/RP. Sometimes, OCD is more tic-like than OCD-like with no obsessions or anxieties to habituate using exposure. The patient may be suffering from one of the OC spectrum disorders, such as trichotillomania or skin picking.

In this chapter, we summarize some special techniques that are helpful for patients with these and other conditions that are not as readily amenable to E/RP. Specific interventions include anxiety management training, thought stopping, satiation, massed practice, habit reversal, and some specific interventions for obsessional slowness. Unlike the interventions described in Part II, which are necessary for just about all patients with OCD, these interventions are supplemental and optional because their targets occur only in some children with the disorder. Without them, treatment might not progress satisfactorily, but they are not necessary in the majority of cases.

First, however, a word of warning. As discussed in the preceding chapter, a multiplicity of symptoms may be associated with mental disorders other than OCD. For each symptom constellation there are cognitive-behavioral treatments that cannot be covered in this chapter, but which may be central to the successful treatment of your patient (Clarkin & Kendall, 1992). For example, depressed OCD patients may benefit from cognitive-behavioral treatments for depression. OCD patients with other comorbid anxiety disorders, such as social phobia, generalized anxiety disorder, or panic disorder, will benefit from partial implementation of treatments for these other conditions if the symptoms are interfering with the treatment of OCD or, simply, if they bother the patient. For example, a child with panic-like anxiety during E/RP for OCD may benefit from an intervention that helps the child habituate to dizziness (spinning a chair, for example) or suffocation anxiety (sucking air through a cocktail straw), depending on the particular symptoms that trouble the youngster. Instructions for obtaining the treatment protocols we use to target these comorbid symptoms are provided in Appendix III.

## ANXIETY MANAGEMENT TRAINING

Anxiety management training (AMT) includes specific strategies for managing somatic/autonomic symptoms (breathing training, relaxation training) plus anxiety-reducing imagery strategies that the child can use during E/RP tasks. AMT is useful for those children who become so tense and anxious during E/RP that they invariably "bail out," thereby preventing habituation from occurring. While most children don't require either relaxation or breathing training, those that do are much less likely to engage in escape–avoidance maneuvers during E/RP if these strategies are available. We generally introduce all three strategies—breathing training, relaxation training, and imagery—and combine them as appropriate with the short form of cognitive training to meet the needs of the individual child. AMT may require an extra session, usually following either Session 2 or 3.

### Breathing Training

When tense, many children tend to tighten the diaphragm, which confines breathing to the upper chest so that it feels impossible to "catch your breath." In turn, the sensation of restricted breathing becomes an interoceptive cue that provokes further anxiety. This effect clearly overlaps with symptoms of panic/separation anxiety disorder (Barlow, 1992) and, in young persons with OCD, often accompanies panic-level anxiety, if not panic disorder itself.

To illustrate this effect, the therapist demonstrates diaphragmatic breathing by showing the youngster how the therapist's stomach pushes outward when inhaling and inward when exhaling. The therapist then demonstrates that the opposite thing happens to breathing when the child is anxious. The child is then asked to practice—placing one hand on the stomach just above the navel and one hand on the chest—so that he too can experience the difference. In this way, the child can feel which muscles are sequentially involved in breathing in and out. The therapist then instructs the child to breathe in slowly through the nose and count one, then blow out slowly, saying "relax" to him- or herself. The child practices this several times; the therapist may assist by counting and saying "relax" for the child at an appropriate pace. If the child is having a difficult time using the diaphragm, a helpful exercise is to ask the child (again with hands placed as noted above) to take a breath and say the words "ha, ha, ha" (it is impossible to say "ha" without using the diaphragm). After the child has located the diaphragm, it is helpful to ask the child to first exhale while gently pushing in on the diaphragm. Next the child inhales slowly through the nose (as noted above), allowing the diaphragm to extend outward again. Assure the child that this takes practice and does not come easily at first. It may be helpful to suggest that the child exhale toward his bottom, "kind of like a wave." Younger children sometimes enjoy blowing bubbles to practice blowing out. When first learning to breathe in this way, the child may wish to practice while lying down. In this position, a soft object can be placed on the abdomen and the child can watch the object rise when he inhales and fall when he exhales. In order to slow breathing down (especially when anxious), the child is asked to hold his breath for three counts before slowly exhaling by blowing the air out. The therapist may want to make the analogy with how basketball players at the foul line do this kind of breathing before taking a shot. When the child can demonstrate the ability to breathe with the diaphragm, it is time to introduce deep muscle relaxation training.

## Relaxation Training

While relaxation training has been shown to be an ineffective component of behavioral treatment for OCD in adults (Marks, 1987), it is sometimes helpful with children who become so tense that E/RP is very difficult. The usual format is deep muscle relaxation, which consists of tensing and relaxing large muscle groups in a systematic manner, so that the child eventually learns to relax even under the stress of E/RP.

Relaxation should be taught with the child's active participation, letting him or her try out each step as instructed, and then putting it all together at the end. We first instruct the child to choose a comfortable position, either lying down or sitting up. The therapist then introduces the idea of tensing and then relaxing separate muscle groups, beginning with the neck muscles. Instruct the child to tense the neck muscles by shrugging his shoulders as he counts to five or ten (depending upon the age and needs of the child), and then to slowly relax them by counting backwards to one. Next have the child roll the head, first dropping it forward to rest chin-on-chest, then rolling it to one side, then allowing the head to slowly drop to the back, then to the other side, and again to drop slowly to the front. Repeat this once or twice. The arms follow the neck and are tensed by pulling them forward palms up, again to the same count, and then relaxing them slowly to the backwards count. This tensing and relaxing of muscle groups continues with hands, stomach, legs, and finally feet. These steps may then be repeated working from the feet back up to the head. Have the child practice diaphragmatic breathing at the beginning and end of the exercise.

## Imagery

The final element of AMT involves helping the child relax through imagining a place where he or she enjoys him- or herself and feels relaxed and peaceful. After encouraging the child to imagine a favorite place, the therapist then asks the child to describe all the details of what is imagined—smells, tastes, sights, textures, etc. If the child has difficulty with visualization, imagery scripts in which the therapist guides the experience can help facilitate the child's use of imagination. The subject matter need not be restricted to calm relaxing places, such as the beach or forest, nor does it have to be visual imagery. Music is equally effective for children whose primary sensory preference is auditory rather than visual. Humorous or silly reflections are also appropriate. The important element is that the imagery yields a positive affect conducive to relaxation. When practicing imagery during the session, we usually encourage the child to do so at the end of the deep muscle relaxation, introducing breathing training as well. Note that imagery cannot be used during imaginal exposure tasks, though relaxation and breathing training are appropriate if the child would otherwise not be able to complete the task.

## Short Form

While anxiety-reducing exercises often reduce anxiety in general, the goal of AMT is to provide "tools" for reducing anxiety or other dysphoric affects *during* E/RP tasks. Therefore, it is often more practical to use an abbreviated version of AMT during an E/RP task. In this shortened exercise, the child is instructed to take three or four diaphragmatic breaths then tense and relax both fists and/or feet to the count of 5–10 followed by three or four more breaths, and to repeat the process as needed. It is sometimes helpful for children to picture themselves holding all the anxiety in their fist and letting go of all the anxiety as the fists are relaxed, and then shaking off the last bits of tension by shaking their hands. Once physical anxiety symptoms have come down a bit, the child should also use the self-statements introduced during cognitive training.

Practice the entire sequence of deep breathing and muscle relaxation one time with the child and correct any difficulties, using the fear thermometer to rate the child's anxiety level both before and after relaxation. This reinforces for the child the effect of relaxation on the body. The second practice can take place in the context of an imaginal or in vivo exposure task, using the fear thermometer throughout the task. Ask the child to practice the relaxation exercises each day and to rate the level of anxiety before and after each practice, recording it on the homework sheet. Encourage the child to use these new relaxation tools during exposure tasks.

In using AMT, remember that the goal is not to eliminate anxiety but to make it manageable so that habituation of anxiety can occur during E/RP.

## THOUGHT STOPPING

Thought stopping is a technique that can be used to interrupt and sometimes stop obsessions and mental rituals (Emmelkamp, Bouman, & Scholing, 1989). The technique, which is simple to implement, involves jerking attention off OCD by introducing a powerful competing stimulus. Thought stopping has two basic components: (1) loudly shouting "Stop!" to oneself, while (2) simultaneously snapping a rubber band once against the left wrist. The purpose of this somewhat unusual practice is to momentarily "startle the brain" and interrupt the obsessive thought, so that the child can interject the "tool kit" strategies. For example, immediately following the "Stop," the child might tell herself that her brain is playing tricks on her again and that the worry thoughts she is experiencing are unimportant and can safely be ignored. Next, she would engage her mind on something to compete with the obsessive thought, such as a long math problem, remembering a recipe, or reading a funny story. After the obsession has been interrupted, the child should then implement his or her standard cognitive strategies since the usually momentary distraction offered by thought stopping will not offer complete respite from OCD. If the obsession returns, the process is repeated until the obsession ends.

When practicing thought stopping, a child can sometimes become frustrated from trying so hard to push the thought away. The therapist should encourage the child not so much to push the thought away (as if they were trying to push an elephant), but rather to naturally allow the OCD thoughts to recede in preference to other thoughts that readily take up the time and space previously occupied by OCD. A helpful analogy is allowing the obsession to remain as "background noise," which can eventually be "tuned out" as the child sets his or her thoughts on something else. The alternative thoughts should engage attention easily and should not simply be an attempt on the child's part to tell him- or herself to stop thinking the obsession. Sometimes a repetitive alternative thought can be used, much like a meditative mantra or prayer. Some children have found singing or rapping to be effective thought replacements. Songs or thoughts that illicit humorous or loving feelings are especially powerful, since they replace not only the obsession but also the affect that accompanies it. It is best if children adapt their own preferences and interests for use in this thought stopping tool.

When teaching thought stopping, it is sometimes useful to model it by asking the child to think an obsessive thought, then shouting "Stop!" while clapping your hands. The natural result is replacement of OCD by alarm. In this way, the child actually experiences the startle-associated interruption of the obsessive thought. Follow this procedure immediately with conversation about a specific topic such as a sports team or TV program the child likes, or questions about what he or she ate for dinner the previous day. Of course, the level of startle should be kept reasonable, and the procedure should be explained to the child before the demonstration.

## SATIATION

Although obsessions are themselves an aversive stimulus that ought to be amenable to habituation, in practice they prove difficult to approach (Neziroglu & Neuman, 1990). Satiation is an exposure-based method for habituating obsessions. In satiation, the obsession is prescribed to the child for increasingly longer periods of time. For example, the child might be instructed to call up (or think) the obsession for 15–20 minutes. In this way, the child satiates (or becomes bored with) the obsession. As described in Chapter 8, satiation is sometimes accomplished using a 1-minute closed-loop audiotape (like those used in telephone answering machines). Ask your patient to write down his or her obsessions verbatim as they enter the mind. After the obsessions are written down, ask the patient to record them on the audiotape in your presence, making his or her tone of her voice match the feelings that accompany the obsession as much as possible. For example, the child who has a fear of dying would describe the feared outcome in great detail as though it was actually happening. Schedule a 30–45 minute session once a day during which the patient listens to the audiotape over and over (using a portable tape player with headphones, such as a Sony Walkman) and attempts to generate as much distress as possible. Since pure obsessions are rare, most obsessions in patients who have OCD thoughts only are followed by mental rituals. It is therefore crucial to block these rituals so that obsessional anxiety habituates. In some children, this requires the therapist to actively lead the patient through the satiation procedure (which can then be taped) so that therapist-assisted response prevention disallows avoiding or neutralizing rituals. As always, it is important to engage the child in the decision to use satiation, and to choose targets from the transition zone so that stimuli are presented according to the symptom hierarchy and are therefore tolerable.

## MASSED PRACTICE

Massed practice is similar to satiation except that it is the compulsion that is practiced until performing it loses any sense of urgency. Massed practice is especially useful for those children who have "just so" compulsions. Take, for example, the child who must tap symmetrically—two taps on the right and two taps on the left. This compulsion would be practiced for a set period, say 4 minutes, interposed with brief rest periods of perhaps 1 minute, until reactive inhibition (an almost sensorial diminution of the urge to perform the behavior) occurs. This typically takes 30–45 minutes, although it can be a short as 10 minutes or as long as an hour and a half. Daily practice continues until the child no longer experiences the compulsion spontaneously in his or her daily life. The same guidelines apply to massed practice and satiation, with the child choosing which symptoms to practice. Even embarrassing compulsions may be addressed in this way because the child can choose a time and place to practice, which in turn decreases embarrassment. Conversely, compulsions that depend on environmental triggers or support, such as staring rituals or reassurance seeking, respectively, are not likely to be amenable to massed practice.

## HABIT REVERSAL

Negative affects, such as anxiety, guilt, or disgust, predict compulsions, such as washing in response to contamination fears that respond nicely to E/RP. Not all OCD symptoms involve negative affects, however. Some OCD patients, particularly those whose symptoms are on the boundary with the tic disorders, exhibit "sensory incompleteness" (i.e., the feeling that an action has to be completed "enough" or "just so") as the driving affect. This is often accompanied by stereotypic repeating rituals (Rasmussen & Eisen, 1992). Other patients experience tic-like repeating rituals that are urge-driven. A few have self-directed aggressive obsessions, such as the urge to cut oneself or to break or bend something, that are very difficult to tolerate or for which exposure is clearly inappropriate.

For those patients in whom OCD resembles a complex tic-like repeating ritual, habit reversal procedures, such as those described for trichotillomania or Tourette syndrome (Baer, 1992; Vitulano, King, Scahill, & Cohen, 1992), can sometimes be helpful alone or in combination with response prevention. In habit reversal, patients and their families are taught thought stopping, visualization, relaxation, competing motoric responses, and relapse prevention strategies. Although habit reversal is in wide use in anxiety programs in subspecialty clinics, these procedures have received little empirical attention for disorders other than trichotillomania. Children and adolescents with trichotillomania often use this technique to decrease compulsive hair pulling; however, the technique is applicable to many OCD symptoms that are more urge-driven than phobic in nature (Peterson, Campise,

& Azrin, 1994). Here we use the example of trichotillomania to teach the technique.

Habit reversal begins much like thought stopping, with the child telling him- or herself to "Stop!", while at the same time snapping a rubber band lightly on the whichever wrist the child uses to perform the dreaded ritual or behavior. Next, the child is instructed to clench his fists for a full 2 minutes, while the urge to pull is abating. Technically, fist clenching is termed a "competing response," and was originally intended to activate the opposite muscles to those used in the ritual (Peterson et al., 1994). For example, hair pulling involves flexor/pinching motor activity; the competing response is then to extend the elbow and wrist and to splay the fingers. In practice, any alternative motor activity is sufficient in most cases. For example, it is often possible to use alternative competing responses, such as sitting on the hands, drawing, or playing piano, that are not as obvious as fist clenching or finger splaying. Such discrete alternative competing responses are more likely to be done by the child. The important element in the competing motor response is that the same muscles used to pull (or wash, or erase) must be used in an alternative acceptable activity. When performing the competing response, it is important that the child "compete" for at least 2–5 minutes at a time so that the urge has ample time to attenuate. Since this strategy does not work immediately, it must be practiced. A better name for the technique might be "habit replacement" because, in a sense, that is exactly what the child is doing—replacing an undesirable habit with a more desirable one. The child is instructed to practice the competing response each day as well as each time the undesirable habit occurs, so that gradually the habit is reversed. Of course, the competing response must be something that the child feels comfortable doing.

When implementing competing responses, the therapist should consider three things: gratification, setting, and awareness. First, treatment will vary depending on whether the compulsive behavior occurs in response to an urge and produces gratification, either in the form of tension reduction or actual pleasure. Second, the habit must be "mapped out" so that triggers are understood and can be addressed in treatment. Third, it is important to understand the degree to which the child is aware of both the triggers and the resultant "habit." With typical phobic OCD symptoms (e.g., germ fears), the child usually performs the compulsions consciously in response to the obsession. However, the child with brief tapping or touching compulsions may perform these actions without awareness because the compulsion is more or less automatic. Similarly, the child with trichotillomania may be completely oblivious to the hair pulling until it is finished. Many children fall between these two extremes, performing compulsions automatically and without resistance, but with some awareness of the behavior.

Habits that occur in response to urges must be blocked at the trigger stage or through one of the several response prevention techniques outlined here. Where tension reduction is an issue, other means must be found to address the primary issue of dysphoric affect. For example, if the habit occurs when the patient is stressed or angry, interventions to reduce stress or increase the ability to cope with anger are appropriate. Similarly, if the habit provides an element of gratification or pleasure, it is helpful if the competing response also provides gratification. For example, a young boy who bites his knuckles might use "Tic Tac" candy along with a fiddle toy in order to compete with the urge to bite his finger. The young girl with trichotillomania and root eating rituals might suck on a gumdrop while clenching her fists or drawing. Children and their parents often worry that the competing response will become a new compulsion; however, this is unlikely since the competing response is entirely voluntarily. Nevertheless, it is necessary to choose competing habits that do not interfere substantially with the child's functioning.

The second important consideration involves mapping out where the habit takes place. In this way the child can "red flag" those places and situations that are likely to trigger the habit. Mapping involves monitoring the habit, which can be frustrating for the child because he or she often wants to "just get rid of the habit now!" The child must be encouraged, however, to complete this part of habit reversal because it is necessary to know all about the habit so that the child and therapist together can develop a plan of action. Mapping involves a detailed understanding of where and under what circumstances the habit occurs (and where it does not), as well as of associated thoughts, feelings, and bodily sensations. For example, an adolescent girl who consciously plucks her hair discovers that she often pulls in her room when studying but not when watching TV, and that the pulling is much worse when she is feeling nervous or stressed about her workload. Because she hates the cosmetic consequences of trichotillomania, she spends more time watching TV than studying, which in turn increases her level of stress when she sits down to do her school work. In this instance, hair pulling serves a clear tension-reduction function. Further questioning reveals that pulling does not occur when she is working at the computer—she is using her hands for something else—but does occur absent-mindedly when she is reading, even when she is not stressed. The context of the hair pulling in this second situation is much different, so the intervention will be depend on anticipating the trigger rather than addressing the issue of tension reduction.

For virtually all children, habit reversal involves some element of increasing awareness of triggers; for many, increasing awareness of the habit itself is important. Thus, the third consideration involves determining whether the habit occurs more consciously or unconsciously (i.e., the child's level of awareness before and during the habit). To increase awareness, we use self-monitoring strategies in which the child is asked to use a diary to keep track of the habit. For example, the child might be asked to record where hair pulling occurred and the number of hairs pulled. Recording strategies are useful for initial mapping, as a treatment intervention, and for monitoring the outcome of treatment. Inventiveness is the key to treatment, especially of automatic habits. For example, one young girl who pulled her hair put Band-Aids on her fingers as a way of increasing her awareness. Another young woman tied a rubber band from her belt to her wrist or put perfume on her hand to increase her awareness of moving her hand toward her hair. These devices should not be punitive or embarrassing in any way, since an increase in anxiety usually causes an increase in the habit's occurrence.

Once the gratification, setting, and awareness associated with the habit are understood, the child and therapist can together develop a plan for reversing or replacing the habit. This plan might include not only competing motor responses, but also strategies for reducing generalized stress and anxiety, techniques for increasing awareness, and specific plans for each "red flagged" area where the habit occurs. It may be necessary to have several different plans depending on where and when the habit is occurring. Nighttime pulling before sleep may be handled differently from pulling during study hall. It is often helpful to have the child write these plans down, like a "battle" or "game" plan. Throughout the process of teaching habit reversal, it is vital that the child not feel pressured to change or stop the unwanted habit. Habit reversal requires much patience and practice. It is not a speedy technique and both parents and children often need to be encouraged not to give up hope. The old habit was formed over many months or even years; in the same way, the new more adaptive responses will require a long time to become second nature.

Relapse prevention is also a key element in habit reversal. Brief bursts of self-injurious habits, such as nail biting, cutting or picking, or hair pulling, can do as much damage in a few minutes as was prevented over the preceding several weeks. Such habit flares often occur in response to an external stressor, such as a fight with a loved one, including parents or peers, or anticipating either a welcome event (e.g., a school dance) or a dreaded one (e.g., the SATs). When a particular trigger regularly destroys months of hard work, that trigger then becomes a target for intensive intervention. The most common situation in which such an intervention is called for involves parent–child conflict and hair pulling. In this instance, behavioral family therapy is sometimes necessary to eliminate the hair pulling entirely.

## INTERVENTIONS FOR OBSESSIONAL SLOWNESS

Obsessional slowness (OS) is a relatively uncommon variant of OCD in which patients have difficulty initiating goal-directed action and suppressing perseverative behaviors. Consequently, these patients typically exhibit extreme slowness in the execution of everyday tasks, such as washing, grooming, or eating. Patients with OS may be neurologically more impaired than the average OCD patient (Hymas, Lees, Bolton, Epps, & Head, 1991). The time-consuming repeating rituals may or may not be connected with phobic anxiety, sensory incompleteness, or pathological doubt (Tallis & de Silva, 1992). While some adult OS patients exhibit Parkinsonian-like bradykinesia (e.g., very very slow motor movements like the Tin Man in the *Wizard of Oz*), most children with OS engage in repeating rituals, sometimes for hours on end. It is thus the delay in completing the task, and not the motor activity itself, which makes them "slow." Such children shower, comb their hair, open a drawer, count, touch, or arrange something over and over in response to an urge do so, phobic concerns, or a vague sense of discomfort if the behavior is terminated "prematurely." Rather than rush through rituals to get them completed, they mindlessly repeat the ritualized behavior, sometimes without seeming concerned about the excessive time being consumed by the ritual.

Like adults, most children and adolescents with OS do poorly with E/RP (Foa & Emmelkamp, 1983). As a result, many cognitive-behavioral therapists use therapist-assisted modeling, shaping, limit setting, and temporal speeding procedures with these patients (Ratnasuriya, Marks, Forshaw, & Hymas, 1991). Unfortunately, when therapist assistance is withdrawn, rapid relapse is the rule (Wolff & Rapoport, 1988). Although Clark successfully treated a 13-year-old boy with obsessional slowness using shaping procedures (Clark, 1982), most clinicians and researchers agree that treatment of this subtype of OCD in both adults and youth is ripe for cognitive-behavioral innovation (March, Johnston, & Greist, 1990).

## Modeling and Shaping

Modeling, defined as demonstrating more appropriate or adaptive behaviors, is frequently used during therapist-assisted E/RP. Modeling can be overt (i.e., the child understands that the therapist is providing a demonstration) or covert (i.e., the therapist informally models a behavior). In patients with OS, the therapist simply demonstrates the ordinary behavior and then asks the patient to do the same. For example, a patient who brushes her hair for hours might be asked to do so for 5 minutes. As always, modeling E/RP works only if the child assents. Some children with OS also have intercurrent mental rituals, such as counting, that must be included in the E/RP procedure.

Closely related to modeling, shaping consists of positively reinforcing successive approximations to the target behavior. For example, an AIDS-phobic child might receive positive reinforcement (with praise, if not tangible rewards) for coming closer and closer to an HIV-positive person before finally shaking hands (shaping/exposure), an action that he has seen the therapist take without harm on previous occasions (overt or covert modeling). With children, modeling helps reduce anticipatory anxiety as well as providing an opportunity for cognitive strategizing (Thyer, 1991).

## Slow Mindful Repetition

Slowness rituals are generally conducted automatically. While patients report attending closely to their compulsions, they in fact direct very little attention to the cognitive aspects of motor intention (defined as the "willing it to happen" component of a motor action) or to the visual or sensorimotor cues accompanying their motor rituals. Rather, attention is directed to imagined consequences, accompanying affects and their hoped for resolution, and to the cognitions that accompany these cognitive–emotional processes. For example, a child might report that, while inserting and removing a plug over and over for hours, he or she was attending to the act of manipulating the plug. However, functional analysis of the behavior will show that the child was actually attending to thoughts about the house burning down and/or other cognitive–emotional–physical indicators of anxiety, or perhaps even to something, such as school, entirely unrelated to OCD. In OS patients without phobic anxiety, a similar process occurs. For example, a child may absent-mindedly brush her hair for hours, each time counting to 87, and then starting over until the "enough feeling" arrives and she can move on.

Foa and Wilson described the process of intentionally slowing down rituals as a means of response prevention, but they did not connect the procedure to OS nor did they focus on the cognitive or attention-training aspect of the procedure (Foa & Wilson, 1991). Independently, we developed a cognitive-behavioral technique for OS-associated repeating rituals, which we call slow mindful repetition (SMR). SMR involves training patients to pay mindful attention to motor intention and sensorimotor cues while very slowly performing a single repetition of a chosen ritual. Recall that these patients say that they are paying attention to their rituals, but in fact they are focusing on catastrophic thinking or are even daydreaming while counting absentmindedly. SMR interrupts this process in the following ways:

1. Patients are taught to recognize that they are not, in fact, paying attention to what is actually happening but rather are lost in thoughts spawned by OCD.

2. Patients are taught to closely monitor their thoughts, feelings, and behaviors without necessarily reacting to them. In this form of attention training, patients are instructed to note on a moment-by-moment basis what is happening cognitively, affectively, and motorically (Foa, Rothbaum, & Kozak, 1989). In this way, they are taught to pay attention to what is actually present rather than remaining lost in OCD thoughts. The child simply notes that something—an affect, a sensation, or a thought—has arisen within the attentional field and recognizes that whatever is present will inevitably depart. This aspect of SMR is identical to the intervention for cultivating detachment that we discussed in the section on cognitive training in Chapter 6.

3. Patients are then taught a meditation technique for paying close attention to motor movement and sensorimotor feedback that we adapted from the Vipassana practice of walking meditation (Goleman, 1976; Miller, Fletcher, & Kabat-Zinn, 1995). In walking meditation, the meditator walks very slowly, paying close attention to the

intention to move and to the sensorimotor cues that provide feedback that movement is actually taking place. In order to maximize fine-grained attention, the act of walking is performed very slowly. For example, it is not unusual to take 20 minutes to walk 10 or 15 feet, or, in another application of the same technique, to take 2 or 3 minutes to take a sip of tea. In the treatment of OS, patients are taught to pay close attention to the motor intention and sensorimotor cues accompanying a particular ritual while performing one repetition of the ritual extremely slowly. Response prevention is built in to the procedure by having the patient walk away from the ritual after completing the single repetition.

The key to this form of treatment lies not in the emphasis on RP, but in the awareness practice that precedes it. The procedure is thus developmentally better suited to older children and adolescents who have the cognitive ability and patience to tolerate the inevitable dysphoric affects and distractions that occur.

## SUMMARY

While the interventions described in Part II of this manual will be sufficient for most patients with OCD, a minority either will not benefit or will show only a partial response. For these patients, many of whom have tic-like OCD symptoms, obsessive slowness, or prominent physical anxiety symptoms, adjunctive pharmacotherapeutic or psychotherapeutic interventions will be necessary. The inventive therapist can make headway with many stalled patients by introducing techniques such as thought stopping, anxiety management training, habit reversal, and, for obsessional slowness, modeling/shaping and SMR. To learn more about these interventions, readers should refer to the pertinent readings in the resource list in Appendix III.

# Chapter 19

## Working
## with Families

Family dysfunction does not cause OCD, but families nonetheless affect and are affected by a child with OCD (Lenane, 1989). Typical concerns include control struggles surrounding rituals, difficulty dealing with sexual or aggressive obsessions, and differences of opinion about how to deal with OCD symptoms. Adolescents occasionally find rituals an effective weapon in the struggle for separation and can be reluctant to give them up, even at the expense of individuation. As in schizophrenia, high "expressed emotion" may be an important family mediating variable, with angry affects and hypercritical attitudes exacerbating OCD (Hibbs, Hamburger, Kruesi, & Lenane, 1993). In addition, OCD typically unsettles the family's social and community interactions, including those with health care professionals who may or may not understand the disorder (Hand, 1988).

Some therapists prefer to work with parents; others prefer to leave them in the waiting room. In our view, parents are on the same team with the child and therapist in helping write OCD out of the child's (and the parent's) story. Consequently, graded parent involvement based on a functional analysis of the need to involve family members in treatment is an essential part of the therapeutic process. In this chapter, we present our method for working with families, recognizing that research on this topic is sparse at best (March, 1995; Van Noppen, Steketee, McCorkle, & Pato, 1997).

187

## OCD TANGLES UP FAMILIES TOO

While OCD often causes family troubles and families may or may not cope skillfully with OCD, families are not responsible for causing the disorder. Rather family members typically find themselves having to respond to OCD, much as the child does, since it is possible for OCD to influence family members in ways similar to the influence OCD holds over the child with the disorder. A child's discomfort arises in direct response to OCD; the parent's discomfort is a response to the child's symptoms. If the parent responds by complying with OCD, then the parent unwittingly takes the side of OCD. Conversely, if the parent assists the child with E/RP, OCD loses and the child wins. Take, for example, the youngster who becomes extremely anxious if she is not given clothes that were just removed from the dryer. Her mother may choose to alleviate her daughter's anxiety by washing and drying clean clothes for her every morning (i.e., by becoming entangled in the ritual). A better choice might be for her mother to refuse to do extra laundry, instead requiring her daughter to do it, if she must. When children with OCD must perform the rituals themselves, the desire to be rid of OCD naturally increases, because OCD is such a nuisance. How to engineer this collaborative resistance to OCD is the topic of this chapter.

OCD typically traps family members out of sympathy (e.g., parents naturally wish to ease a child's evident suffering) or out of coercion (e.g., OCD may cause a child such distress that he or she demands parental compliance with the rituals), or simply out of ignorance (OCD doesn't come with an owner's guide, and parents, like their children, may not know how best to respond to it). The risk of parental involvement in rituals also seems to vary according to the degree of discomfort that the parent experiences in response to the child's OCD symptoms, especially when the parent also suffers from OCD, another anxiety disorder, or depression. Under these circumstances, parents who are very involved with the child's rituals and/or have OCD/anxiety symptoms themselves need special support, understanding, and encouragement at the beginning of treatment (March, 1995; Piacentini, Gitow, Jaffer, & Graae, 1994). Not all families start out with a supportive attitude toward their children, who may themselves show disruptive behaviors apart from OCD. When parents are at odds over how best to respond to OCD, it is often best to focus first on finding ways to decrease parental distress (Steketee, 1994). When this is impossible, and family or marital conflict is interfering with the treatment of OCD, then marital or family therapy may be appropriate.

## ASSESSING FAMILY INVOLVEMENT IN OCD

Assessing OCD in the family context is complex, since it involves several overlapping dimensions, each of which has the potential to help or hinder treatment. At the most basic level, psychoeducation into the nature of the disorder and the nature of the treatment program is essential for all families. The therapist should also consider the extent to which OCD involves family members, how the developmental stage of the child affects family relations, the potential for parents to help with treatment, and the presence of negative family interactions.

### Extent to Which OCD Involves Family Members

Clearly, the extent to which OCD traps other people besides the child dictates their involvement in treatment. When OCD involves only the child, and the family is otherwise supportive, family involvement can safely be minimized. When OCD has a dramatic influence on one or more family members, their participation in treatment is mandatory. Therefore, the systematic assessment of triggers, avoidance behaviors, obsessions, and rituals *as they involve other people* is a necessary part of establishing a stimulus hierarchy.

### Developmental Stage

Younger children, particularly those in preschool or early elementary years, are more dependent on parents for a variety of activities in their daily lives. Adolescents may be ready and willing to direct their own treatment independently of parents; however, OCD may be bound up in control struggles between the young adult and parents or teachers. Early adolescents especially don't like to be different from their peers with whom they identify strongly. Thus, they are sometimes embarrassed not only by their OCD symptoms but also by having their parents involved in their treatment. Not surprisingly then, the child's developmental stage dramatically influences the extent to which parents can become (as differentiated from need to become) involved in treatment. To the extent that the child functions independently, needing relatively little guidance from parents with respect to daily activities and OCD, the focus can remain on individual treatment. When the converse is true—for example, because of younger age, cognitive limitations, or severe functional impairment—the need for family involvement increases.

## Potential for Parental Helpfulness

All families should be encouraged to eliminate punishment for OCD, minimize unnecessary advice giving, and differentially reinforce other positive behaviors. Beyond these most basic interventions, the extent to which parents can and wish to become constructively involved in treatment is an important issue to raise with parents and children. At the beginning of treatment, the therapist should determine the expectations of both parent and child in this regard and check these expectations against the capacity of the parent to help and of the child to make use of parental assistance. Even when it isn't essential, parents can be very helpful by providing ample support and encouragement or, in some cases, by becoming a lay cotherapist as the child resists OCD.

## Identifying Negative Family Interactions

Ideally, families should behave in a loving and supportive manner toward a child who is ill with OCD. In reality, more than a few families exhibit an enduring pattern of negative interactions that exacerbate OCD and threaten the progress of CBT. Such negative interactions typically take four forms: (1) negative interactions related to OCD itself, (2) negative family interactions related to activities of daily living, (3) sibling issues, and (4) marital conflict. Each type of interaction can be exacerbated by a family member's intercurrent mental illness. If this is the case, the illness of the family member must be sensitively identified and treated where necessary (usually by referring the affected parent or sibling to an appropriate resource). Negative family interactions related to OCD are easily identified when mapping the disorder. Negative family interactions related to other activities are a bit harder to identify, but often emerge in the confusion between parent and child over what is or is not related to OCD. Trouble with siblings often occurs because of sibling rivalry, especially when the ill child is getting most of the attention, or because OCD has the sibling tangled up or seriously inconvenienced by rituals. Finally, when parents disagree over OCD—with one parent playing "good cop" (emphasizing comfort and consolation) and the other playing "bad cop" (emphasizing punishment)—the resultant conflict very often constrains the therapist's ability to implement the CBT treatment program and must be addressed in treatment.

## LEVEL OF FAMILY INVOLVEMENT IN TREATMENT

Fortunately, the great majority of children and adolescents with OCD do very well with individual CBT. When it is not needed, intensive family involvement often leads to resentment and noncompliance with treatment. Conversely, when the clinical situation requires it, the failure to graduate from individual CBT to more intensive family-based treatment strategies may seriously limit the potential benefits of CBT for OCD. Grading family involvement according to clinical exigencies therefore requires a careful and thoughtful assessment of OCD, comorbidities, and family functioning as well as sensitive communication with parents regarding their involvement in treatment. More often than not, we begin with individual CBT, with adjunctive parental involvement, and graduate to greater parental involvement as need dictates. Less commonly, when the initial evaluation clearly demonstrates that individual work is likely to founder on the shoals of family psychopathology, we involve parents in greater depth from the beginning. As shown in Table 19.1, which presents appropriate levels of family involvement in treatment based on the child's developmental stage, need for extinction strategies, the potential of the

**TABLE 19.1.** Dimensions to Consider in Assessing the Need for Family Involvement in Treatment

| Dimension | Level of family involvement in treatment | | | |
|---|---|---|---|---|
| | Primarily individual CBT | Mix of individual and family sessions | CBT primarily in the family setting | Individual and concurrent behavioral family therapy |
| Child's developmental stage | Older age | Any age | Younger age | Usually older age |
| Need for extinction strategies | Less | More | Extensive | Varies |
| Potential for family helpfulness | Yes | Yes | Yes | Limited at start |
| Destructive family interactions | If not present | If mild | If moderate | If severe |

family to be helpful, and the presence of destructive family interactions, family work in treatment typically takes one of the following
forms:

- *Primarily individual CBT.* Over 90% of our patients are successfully treated with a model that focuses primarily on the child, with
parents, siblings, and other adults serving the important but adjunctive
role of ally in the child's struggle against OCD. In this model, which
was described in detail in Part II of this manual, parents participate
fully in specific sessions, including sessions devoted to education and
implementation of extinction strategies, and for a few minutes at the
beginning and end of all other sessions. Otherwise, the contest between OCD and the child primarily involves helping the child learn
and implement a successful strategy for resisting OCD. This is the most
common strategy, which provides for family support, knowledge building, and reduced participation in rituals.

- *Mix of family and individual CBT.* In this option, several extra
family sessions are necessary to address disentangling family members
from involvement in rituals, reducing family conflicts that may be
interfering with CBT for OCD, or helping parents structure more
intensive involvement in treatment as cotherapists. For example,
John Piacentini at the University of California at Los Angeles
(Piacentini et al., 1994) and Anne Marie Albano at the University
of Louisville (Albano, Knox, & Barlow, 1995) have shown that
concurrent family work is especially useful when extinction strategies
play a major role in treatment. To encourage parents to pay attention
to and reinforce pleasing family interactions and to discourage
negative family interactions, we typically rely on differential reinforcement of other behavior (DRO) and on reinforcement of incompatible behavior (RIB). DRO depends on extinction (systematically
ignoring problem behaviors) while simultaneously reinforcing more
adaptive behaviors. RIB involves substituting a more adaptive for a
less adaptive behavior in the same domain of functioning. For
example, a parent might ignore reassurance seeking concerning
contamination themes (extinction) while paying more attention to
school work (DRO) and emphasizing a greater frequency of chores
involving appropriate cleaning (RIB). Both DRO and RIB implicitly
foster response prevention.

- *CBT as family therapy.* When OCD severely tangles up family
members, or when the patient is a preschool age child for whom
parental involvement in most aspects of the child's life is the rule

rather than the exception, CBT is best done in the context of continuous family involvement in treatment. In this situation, the CBT program is the same as in individual therapy; the only difference is that one or both parents are present for the duration of each session.

• *Behavioral family therapy.* Finally, some families are so thoroughly tangled up in OCD, so bedeviled by accompanying comorbidities, such as a disruptive behavior disorder, or show such significant family dysfunction, that individual CBT is impossible (Wells, 1995). When this turns out to be the case, behavioral family therapy, including formal parent training, plus individual CBT for the child are indicated. In the most intensive variation on this theme, the child's individual therapist accompanies the patient to the family sessions, which are conducted by a different therapist, thereby avoiding the problem of the divided loyalties that may be engendered when a single therapist attempts CBT for OCD and behavioral contracting at the same time. As commonly, individual CBT is deferred until family therapy—conducted by a separate family therapist—allows individual CBT to begin while concurrent family therapy continues.

## FOLLOWING THE CHILD'S LEAD

Irrespective of the level of family involvement, tackling OCD at the child's own pace is a therapeutic priority that should be violated only when dangerousness arises or child or family dysfunction is so severe that it must be addressed immediately (e.g., a child who is cutting him- or herself, defecating all around the house, or refusing to attend school). Generally though, it is important to use the transition/work zone as a guide for E/RP tasks involving parents, teachers, or siblings. Doing so requires considerable patience, since rituals that involve parents are not uncommonly located deep in OCD's territory, and so are not found in the transition zone at the beginning of treatment. Rarely, when treatment is stalled and the family is severely bothered by OCD, parents may be encouraged to select targets for response prevention or extinction, even when the child protests. As noted in Chapter 10, such unilateral extinction procedures have significant disadvantages that make it a treatment of last resort. These disadvantages include: (1) parents' lack of a workable strategy for managing the child's distress, (2) disruption of the treatment relationship, (3) parents' inability to target symptoms that are out of the sight of parents and teachers; and, most importantly, (4) the failure of nonconsensual extinction to help the child internalize a more skillful strategy for coping with current and potential future OCD symptoms. Fortunately, all that is needed in most instances is to instruct parents to stop giving unhelpful advice and insisting on inappropriate exposure tasks, while both parents and child learn how to cope more effectively with OCD.

## HAVING OCD HAS MEANING

While the content of obsessions is for the most part best ignored, the meaning attending having a mental illness—in this case, OCD— is of crucial importance to all family members. Children and their families often feel helpless and overwhelmed by OCD, as if all of life was being tainted by the disorder. OCD often skews relations with the medical and school system, as well as with family friends and relatives, in a negative direction. It is therefore important to address the impact of OCD on the child and family in order for treatment to progress and be effective. Many parents and children have questions about the implications of OCD with regard to having children. An excellent booklet by Hugh Johnston, MD, of the University of Wisconsin dealing with such topics related to OCD in young persons is available from the OC Foundation (see "Resources" in Appendix III).

## THE ROLE OF CONTINGENCY MANAGEMENT

It is not possible to treat OCD through a system of rewards and punishments (i.e., by implementing a contingency management procedure). No one hates OCD more than the child who has it; consequently, bribes will be ineffective since the child would stop on her own if she only could. Simply stated, punishment makes OCD worse, and punishing someone for being sick is unreasonable in any event. On the other hand, children and adolescents do not always behave well and it is not always easy to distinguish OCD from behaviors unrelated to OCD, for which rewards or punishment may be appropriate.

Ideally, a simple mutually agreed-upon rubric for distinguishing OCD from everything else is all that is needed. For example, the parents can use the child's nasty nickname for OCD to ask the child whether a particular problematic behavior is related to OCD or not. If the answer is yes, sympathy is the appropriate response; if not, whatever consequences are appropriate to the situation should ensue. The therapist will often want to help negotiate such an arrangement early in treatment. Under some circumstances, it can be helpful to treat E/RP as a chore, for which the child earns a reward. We typically help parents set up a developmentally appropriate token or reward system that targets the child's faithful completion of CBT tasks. Such rewards are not bribes but a recognition by an appreciative parent of the fact that the child is doing an activity that is unpleasant, effortful, and time consuming, just like other chores.

In some cases, children with comorbid disruptive behavior disorders, as well as children who refuse to acknowledge that OCD is problematic, may require a contingency management program to make CBT work. For example, it can be difficult for an active child, much less a youngster with ADHD, to make time each day for E/RP; contingency management can help the child with ADHD remain focused on doing CBT homework. Under these circumstances the therapist should help the parent and child negotiate a "contract" that specifies a minimum level of effort for cooperation.

When secondary gain from OCD is a problem—for example, when OCD, while still annoying, allows the child to escape from unpleasant responsibilities, which other family members then pick up—contingency management may encourage compliance with family responsibilities or, at least, a more equitable division of labor among family members. In this instance, contingency management can be quite useful for the child who sees no overriding value in giving up his or her compulsions, for example, the child who misses her first class every day, which she dislikes anyway, because compulsions slow her down, or the adolescent who has germ fears and consequently is never expected to clean up after himself. In this instance, the child who misses school in the morning might forfeit a certain amount of free play in the afternoon exactly in the same way that a child who is sick would be expected to stay indoors. The avoidant adolescent might be given household responsibilities that do not trigger OCD in order to have access to the car on weekends. Naturally, contingency management programs must be individualized to meet the particular situation of the child and family.

The protocol described in this manual focuses on CBT for OCD and not disruptive behaviors. However, readers will find references to contingency management procedures as well as such useful interventions as anger coping and panic control training in Appendix III.

## SUMMARY

To summarize, we include families in treatment from the very beginning, grading and tailoring family involvement to the particular needs of the child and his or her family. During the first session, families discover together what is meant by putting OCD into a neurobehavioral framework. During Sessions 7 and 12 more intensive parent assessment and intervention is encouraged. During these sessions, we examine how and in what ways OCD is influencing family members and discuss strategies for helping family members resist OCD. Parents are also encouraged to share questions and concerns at the beginning and end of each session; if needed, additional parent sessions may be scheduled at any time. Finally, for families in which OCD or other problems make individual treatment impractical, the CBT protocol outlined in this manual can easily be scaled up to include more intensive family involvement.

Chapter 20

# Working with Schools
## with Gail Adams

Because school personnel have the opportunity to observe and interact with students for several hours a day, they are in a unique position to identify OCD symptoms in school-age children (Adams et al., 1994). School personnel may in fact represent a first line of defense in the identification of OCD. It is critical, therefore, that classroom teachers, school psychologists, counselors, social workers, nurses, and administrators learn to identify OCD symptoms in the school setting, help make appropriate referrals, and assist, as appropriate, in the treatment of childhood OCD. In this chapter, we (1) discuss the signs and symptoms of childhood OCD in the school environment, (2) present suggestions regarding the role of school personnel in the diagnosis and treatment of OCD, and (3) provide suggestions for managing OCD symptoms in the school setting. Although we briefly review the treatment of OCD with CBT and medication, the focus in this chapter is on managing OCD in the school setting.

It may be helpful to copy this chapter for school personnel so that they can learn more about OCD, which will enable them to better ally with the affected child, therapist, and family members in the treatment process.

### RECOGNIZING OCD IN THE SCHOOL SETTING

Because many children and adolescents with OCD are secretive about the disorder, signs of OCD may not be obvious to the casual observer. It is essential that school personnel be aware of and attentive to the symptoms of OCD which are described in the following sections. If unheeded, these symptoms could evolve into a full-blown and more serious expression of the disease that could render the afflicted child unable to attend school. At this late stage, school personnel will have missed the opportunity to help halt the progression of the disorder.

## OBSESSIONS

Obsessions are recurrent and persistent thoughts, impulses, or images that intrude into an individual's thinking. Obsessions are capable of producing tremendous anxiety or feelings of discomfort such as disgust and guilt. Obsessions should be distinguished from the compulsions and mental rituals that an individual may perform in response to an obsession. We describe below some of the more common obsessions exhibited by children and adolescents with OCD.

### Fear of Contamination

Fears of contamination may center around a concern with germs, dirt, ink, paint, excrement, body secretions, blood, chemicals, and other substances. An increase in obsessions with AIDS has recently also become common. Preoccupation with contamination may cause the child or adolescent to avoid suspected contaminants and/or to wash excessively.

### Fear of Harm, Illness, or Death

Children and adolescents with OCD may experience fears of harm, illness, or death. These fears often appear as concern for their own safety or for the safety of significant others. In some cases, young people with OCD are afraid that they will inflict, rather than encounter, harm. They may also be plagued by thoughts of death due to poisoning, germs, and sharp objects.

### Number Obsessions

Obsessions with numbers are particularly common among young boys. Only certain numbers are considered "safe" numbers, while others are "bad." An obsession with a particular number may result in a child having to repeat an action a given number of times (e.g., touching a tree 25 times, striking one's head against the wall 10 times) or having to count repeatedly to a particular number.

## Scrupulosity

Some children and adolescents with strong religious ties have an obsessive fear that they will do something evil. This symptom of OCD, termed "scrupulosity," causes individuals to tell themselves that they consistently commit sins, and that they must therefore pray constantly or find ways to punish themselves for their imagined sins. Some individuals create elaborate systems to avoid certain thoughts, memories, or actions. The obsession that the child might somehow have cheated is particularly common in the school setting.

### BEHAVIORAL MANIFESTATIONS OF OBSESSIONS

Obsessions can be extremely intrusive and may interfere with the normal thinking process. Students experiencing obsessions may get "stuck," or fixated, on certain points, and lose the need or ability to go on. Fixation on a thought may cause distraction from the task at hand, which delays students in completing school work and can lead to a decrease in work production and poor grades. In some cases, a drastic change in academic performance may occur. Whenever a case of school failure or refusal is being evaluated, the possibility of OCD should be considered. It is crucial to note that fixation on an obsessional thought may appear to be and is often mistaken for an attention problem, daydreaming, laziness, or poor motivation.

### COMPULSIONS

Compulsions are repetitive behaviors or mental acts that the person feels driven to perform in response to an obsession or according to rules that must be applied rigidly. Individuals perform these actions or rituals in order to prevent or reduce distress or prevent some dreaded event or situation. Some of the more common compulsions reported by children and adolescents with OCD are described below.

## Washing/Cleaning Rituals

At some point during their illness, approximately 80% of children and adolescents with OCD experience washing or cleaning rituals, the most commonly of which is handwashing. These individuals may feel compelled to wash extensively and according to a self-prescribed manner for minutes to hours at a time. Others may be less thorough about washing or cleaning, but may engage in the act an astounding number of times each day.

Washing and cleaning compulsions may appear in the school setting as subtle behaviors that are not obviously or immediately related to washing or cleaning. For example, students who frequently excuses themselves from the classroom under the guise of voiding may actually be seeking a private place in which to carry out cleaning rituals. Another sign of excessive washing is the presence of dry, red, chapped, cracked, and even bleeding hands. Children have been known to wash with strong cleaning agents (e.g., Mr. Clean) to free themselves of "contaminants."

While contamination fears frequently lead to excessive washing, they may also produce the opposite effect: shoes may be untied, clothing may be slovenly, and hair may be dirty. In these cases, fear of contamination of personal objects or body parts leads to the individual's refusal to touch them. A combination of excessive handwashing and sloppiness in other areas of grooming has even been reported.

## Checking Rituals

Checking rituals are another type of compulsion experienced by youth with OCD. These rituals, which are often precipitated by a fear of harm to self or others, include continual checking of doors, windows, light switches, electrical outlets, water faucets, appliances, and other items. Other children are plagued by pathological doubt rather than a fear of harm. Doubting obsessions (e.g., doubting that a door is actually locked or that an assignment was actually turned in) may be particularly strong.

Checking compulsions can create serious problems for the school-age child. In the process of getting ready for school, a child may check his or her books over and over again to see if all the necessary books are there, even to the point of being late to school. Once in school, the child may feel compelled to call or return home in order to check something yet another time. School personnel should also be alert to rituals such as checking and rechecking answers on assignments to the point that they are submitted late or not at all or repeatedly checking a locker to see if it is locked. Checking rituals may also interfere with the completion of homework—compulsive checking sometimes causes a student to work late into the night on assignments that should have taken 2 or 3 hours to complete.

## Repeating Rituals

Some OCD sufferers who experience feelings that an action has to be completed "enough" or "just so" engage in repeating rituals. In other cases, repeating rituals are driven by anxiety. Individuals with repeating compulsions may walk forward and backward in a particular fashion, get up and down from a chair several times, or go in and out of a doorway in a self-prescribed manner until it "feels right." Repeating rituals are frequently connected with counting rituals in which an action must be repeated a certain number of times.

Repeating rituals may assume many different forms in the classroom, including repetitious questioning, reading and rereading sentences or paragraphs in a book, or sharpening pencils several times in succession. A student experiencing repeating rituals may also endlessly cross out, trace, or rewrite letters or words, or erase and reerase words on a paper until holes are worn in it. Repeating rituals may seriously interfere with a student's ability to take notes, complete computer-scored tests, and even execute lock combinations.

## Symmetry and Exactness Rituals

Obsessions revolving around a need for symmetry may result in a student compulsively arranging objects in the classroom (e.g., books on a shelf, items on a page, pencils on a desk). Symmetry-related rituals may also result in a child feeling compelled to have both sides of his or her body identical (e.g., laces on shoes), to take steps that are identical in length, or to place equal stress on each syllable of a word.

## Other Compulsive Behaviors

OCD sufferers frequently experience obsessional thoughts that lead to compulsive avoidance. In these cases, individuals may go to great lengths to avoid objects, substances, or situations that are capable of triggering fear or discomfort. For example, fear of contamination may cause the child to avoid objects commonly found in the classroom, such as paint, glue, paste, clay, tape, and ink. A child may even inappropriately cover his or her hands with clothing or gloves or use shirttails or cuffs to open doors or turn on faucets. A student with an obsessive fear of harm may avoid using scissors or other sharp tools in the classroom. In a related vein, a child may circumvent the use of a particular doorway because passage through that entry may trigger a repeating ritual.

Children and adolescents with OCD may also engage in compulsive reassurance seeking. For example, in school, they may continually ask teachers or other school personnel for reassurance that there are no germs on the drinking fountain or that they have not made any errors on a page. Obsessions concerning fear of cheating typically cause children to compulsively seek reassurance, avoid looking at other children, and sometimes even to give wrong answers intentionally. Unfortunately, the relief derived from such attempts at reassurance is often short-lived, since different situations continually arise in the classroom that raise new fears or discomfort for the student.

## COMORBID CONDITIONS

It is crucial that school personnel be aware that other disorders frequently co-occur (i.e., are comorbid) with OCD (Adams et al., 1994). For example, anxiety disorders other than OCD (e.g., social phobia) are particularly common among youth with OCD. Adjustment disorders, depression, oppositional defiant disorder, ADHD, and Tourette syndrome may also be seen in conjunction with OCD. Nonverbal learning disorders (LDs) are also common in children with OCD, and LD symptoms (such as poor handwriting, poor math skills, problems with written language, and slow processing speed) may be confused with OCD. The presence of more than one disorder complicates treatment for OCD as well as school management. The remedy is to be clear about the targets of treatment.

## THE ROLE OF SCHOOL PERSONNEL
## IN AN OCD INTERVENTION

### Identification

To successfully identify OCD in the school setting, school personnel must become knowledgeable about OCD in the same way that many now understand LDs or ADHD. Knowledge may be gained by keeping abreast of current information on OCD and by attending lectures and seminars on OCD. School districts are also urged to invite mental health professionals with expertise in OCD to provide in-service training to staff members on institute days or during other professional development periods. Classroom teachers are a particularly critical resource in the identification of OCD given the amount of time they spend with students on a daily basis. They are also in a position to receive verbal reports from students regarding the behavior of a student who exhibits OCD-like behaviors. Teachers can effectively document social and academic problems in the classroom by keeping written records.

Careful assessment is another essential aspect of the identification of school-age children with OCD. When a classroom teacher identifies a student who is possibly exhibiting OCD symptoms, the next step is referral to the school psychologist or student services team. Appropriate team members can then obtain additional information about the student in question. The assessment may include soliciting information from parents, classroom teachers, and the child or adolescent involved.

## Referral

If information derived from the assessment process suggests that a child may have OCD, it is incumbent upon school personnel to meet with the parents, share the results of the team's assessment, and make recommendations for an outside evaluation. School personnel should be familiar with the names of several agencies that are competent in the treatment of childhood OCD.

## Treatment

After a mental health provider diagnoses a child as having OCD, the attending clinician(s) will implement one of several different treatment methods. Cognitive-behavioral therapy, alone or in combination with medication, represents the foundation of treatment for children and adolescents with OCD. Once a treatment program has been established, the student services team should meet with pertinent members of the mental health agency to decide on school-based interventions. For example, an intervention to reduce reassurance seeking or frequent requests to go to the bathroom may be necessary. It will also be important to devise a plan for communicating information among involved parties. Regardless of the treatment intervention selected, a home–school–community partnership is essential in developing and implementing interventions that provide the greatest benefit to students with OCD.

It is important for school personnel to recognize that OCD is a neurobehavioral disorder and that it reflects abnormal information processing in the central nervous system and not "oppositional behavior." School personnel should be encouraged to view the child with OCD in the same fashion as they would a child with a condition such as diabetes or asthma, which can also often cause a child to do poorly until the disease process is arrested and then reversed with treatment. Treatment of OCD, like that of diabetes or asthma, relies on medication (a serotonin reuptake inhibitor) and a psychosocial intervention (cognitive-behavioral therapy), both of which work their magic by acting directly on the brain. Finally, accommodations for what cannot yet be cured are necessary for any chronically ill child, and this is no less true for the child with OCD than it is for the child with asthma or diabetes.

## SUGGESTIONS FOR MANAGING OCD SYMPTOMS IN THE SCHOOL SETTING

School personnel may play an integral role not only in OCD treatment interventions, but also in the daily management of OCD symptoms in the school setting, assuming that such symptoms are present. The following strategies can help school staff facilitate the adjustment of the child or adolescent with OCD to the school setting:

• Refrain from punishing the student for situations or behaviors over which he or she has no control (e.g., being tardy, absent, not attending to work). On the other hand, remember that children with OCD, like all children, have behavior problems that may be helped by setting clear limits and establishing consequences for behavior.

• Be sensitive to the emotional needs of the student with OCD. Children and adolescents with OCD sometimes have low self-esteem and experience trouble with peer relationships, even to the point of being socially isolated. Try to structure class activities so that these students are included. Never tolerate teasing directed toward children or adolescents with OCD. Also consider designating one school employee as the individual to whom the child can turn when he or she is struggling and assigning the student with OCD to a teacher or teachers more empathic to the child's needs.

• Try to be understanding of and provide support to the parents and family of the student with OCD. Families of children with OCD, particularly parents, frequently experience great emotional pain and frustration as they grapple with their child's illness. Therefore, it is important to approach parents with an attitude of caring and concern. Blaming parents for a child's OCD is unwarranted and inappropriate. It is also essential to keep lines of communication open.

• Be attentive to and record changes in a child's behavior (both negative and positive) that may be the result of medication and/or behavioral interventions.

School personnel can also make the following specific changes in the learning environment in order to facilitate the academic performance of students with OCD:

• For the student with OCD who has difficulty taking notes or writing due to writing compulsions, consider accommodations such as tape-recording lectures, providing an outline of the lecture for the student, allowing another student to provide a carbon/photocopy of notes for the student, and permitting the student to put assignments, tests, and homework on the computer or on tape.

• For the student with OCD who has reading compulsions, classroom teachers may tape-record chapters in texts, allow someone else to read to the student, and assign shorter reading assignments to the student.

• For the student with OCD who has difficulty taking tests, the teacher may: (1) allow breaks during testing, (2) provide extra time or a different test-taking location, (3) permit the student to write directly on the test booklet rather than filling in circles on computerized test sheets, and (4) allow the student to take tests orally. Be sure to allow students with OCD to submit assignments or homework after the dates they are due. Also consider decreasing the student's workload. For example, instead of having the child complete all the items on a sheet, have him or her do only the odd or even numbered items or items that have been starred by the teacher.

• While some children with OCD may attempt to use OCD as a crutch to avoid school or schoolwork, most prefer to do their work as best they can. When a child appears to be using OCD as an excuse to avoid classroom or social activities, it is crucial to coordinate the E/RP tasks with the child's cognitive-behavioral therapist so that the teacher knows what to expect of the child with respect to OCD and academically.

## EDUCATIONAL SERVICES FOR CHILDREN AND ADOLESCENTS WITH OCD

The educational needs of children and adolescents with OCD vary tremendously. For some students, symptoms are mild to moderate and may not interfere with academic or social functioning in the school setting, while other students may require only minor adaptations in the learning environment (see above). However, some children and adolescents with more severe cases of OCD may require special education services.

A student with OCD may be eligible for special services under the Individuals with Disabilities Education Act (IDEA) if that child is determined to be a "child with disability" (with OCD, the disability category would be "Other Health Impaired," or, in some school districts, "Serious Emotional Disturbance" LD might also be applicable if the child has a learning disability), and who, by reason thereof, needs special education and related services. Alternatively, under Section 504 of the Rehabilitation Act of 1973, a child may be eligible for services if he/she is determined to be an "individual with a handicap." Section 504 defines an individual with a handicap as one who "has a physical or mental impairment which substantially limits one or more major life activities, has a record of such an impairment, or is regarded as having such an impairment." Major life activities include caring for one's self, peforming manual tasks, walking, seeing, hearing, speaking, breathing, learning, and working. Whether a parent should go with IDEA or Section 504 will depend on a complex mix of factors including parent and school preference, as well as the nature of the youngster's OCD symptoms and other accompanying problems. Working with an OCD-saavy school psychologist often can be invaluable in sorting out the best way to craft an individualized educational plan (IEP) that is appropriate to the educational and social needs for the child or adolescent with OCD.

A psychoeducational assessment may also be needed to evaluate for LDs, which sometimes coexist with OCD. Nonverbal LDs often coexist with OCD and can cause dysgraphia, dyscalculia, and poor expressive written language. Because each of these problems may be a direct reflection of OCD or an indirect result of NVLDs, or a combination of the two, psychoeducational testing is mandatory for the child with OCD who is performing below expectations academically.

## SUMMARY

In summary, OCD is one of the more common mental illnesses affecting children and adolescents. The disorder is not infrequently comorbid with other psychiatric conditions, and may presage adult OCD as well. Treatment is specific to OCD—medications and cognitive-behavioral therapy—and should be administered by a multidisciplinary treatment team familiar with the disorder. School personnel are in a unique position to identify OCD and to participate in pedagogic and behavioral interventions for children and adolescents with this and other childhood-onset anxiety disorders.

# Appendix I

# Handouts and Figures

# Handout 1. Your CBT Program

### What Happens during the Treatment?

| Visit number | Goals |
|---|---|
| Week 1 | Education about OCD<br>Cognitive training |
| Week 2 | Mapping OCD<br>Cognitive training |
| Week 3–18 | Exposure and response prevention |
| Weeks 18–19 | Relapse prevention and graduation |
| Week 24 | Booster session |
| Visits 1, 7, & 12 | Parent sessions |

### What Happens at Each Session?

| Session goals | Time |
|---|---|
| Check in with child and parents | 5 minutes |
| Review homework | 5 minutes |
| Teaching/learning tasks for week | 20 minutes |
| Therapist-assisted practice | 10 minutes |
| Discuss and agree on homework | 10 minutes |
| Parent review of session and homework | 10 minutes |

### What Tools Will You Be Learning?

| Tool | Purpose |
|---|---|
| Externalizing OCD | Making it clear to everyone that OCD is the problem |
| Making allies | Getting everyone on your side |
| Mapping OCD | Understanding where to start "bossing back" OCD |
| Cognitive training | Keeping your thoughts straight about OCD |
| Fear thermometer | Grading OCD from easy to hard to resist |
| Exposure | Facing what you are afraid of |
| Response prevention | Learning how not to do rituals |
| Helping your family | Helping you disentangle family members from OCD |

# Handout 2.  Map Figure

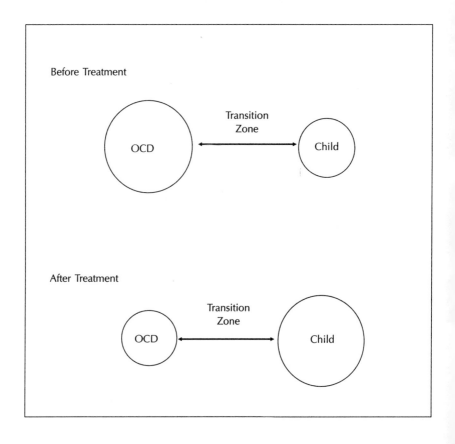

# Handout 3. Fear Thermometer

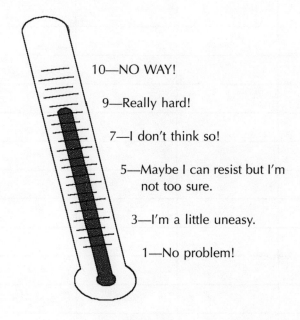

10—NO WAY!

9—Really hard!

7—I don't think so!

5—Maybe I can resist but I'm not too sure.

3—I'm a little uneasy.

1—No problem!

# Handout 4. Symptom List (Stimulus Hierarchy)

| Trigger/situation | Obsession | Compulsion | Temperature (1–10) |
|---|---|---|---|
| | | | |
| | | | |
| | | | |
| | | | |
| | | | |
| | | | |
| | | | |
| | | | |
| | | | |
| | | | |
| | | | |
| | | | |
| | | | |
| | | | |
| | | | |
| | | | |
| | | | |

# Handout 5. Homework Sheet

**E/RP TASKS**

_____

_____

_____

_____

**CLUES TO "BOSSING BACK"**

_____

_____

_____

_____

| Target/ date/ time | Start temp. | 1 min. | 2 mins. | 5 mins. | 10 mins. | 15 mins. | 20 mins. | 25 mins. | 30 mins. |
|---|---|---|---|---|---|---|---|---|---|
| | | | | | | | | | |
| | | | | | | | | | |
| | | | | | | | | | |
| | | | | | | | | | |
| | | | | | | | | | |
| | | | | | | | | | |
| | | | | | | | | | |
| | | | | | | | | | |
| | | | | | | | | | |
| | | | | | | | | | |

# Appendix II

# Assessment Instruments

215

# NIMH Global Obsessive–Compulsive Scale

**Directions:** Circle the number (1 to 15) that best describes the present clinical state of the patient based on the guidelines below:

1  **Minimal within range of normal or very mild symptoms.** Person
2  spends little time resisting them. Almost no or no interference in
3  daily activity.

4  **Subclinical obsessive–compulsive behavior.** Mild symptoms that
5  are noticeable to patient and observer, cause mild interference in
6  patient's life and which he may resist for a minimal period of time.
   Easily tolerated by others.

7  **Clinical obsessive–compulsive behavior.** Symptoms that cause
8  significant interference in patient's life and which he spends a
9  great deal of conscious energy resisting. Requires some help from
   others to function in daily activity.

10  **Severe obsessive–compulsive behavior.** Symptoms that are
11  crippling to the patient, interfering so that daily activity is "an
12  active struggle." Patient may spend full time resisting symptoms.
    Requires much help from others to function.

13  **Very severe obsessive–compulsive behavior.** Symptoms that
14  completely cripple patient so that he requires close staff
15  supervision over eating, sleeping, and so forth. Very minor
    decision making or minimal activity require staff support, "worst
    I've ever seen."

*Source:* National Institute of Mental Health (public domain).

# Clinical Global Impairment Scale

Considering your total clinical experience with this particular problem, how mentally ill is the patient at this time? Circle one (most appropriate).

1 = Normal, not at all ill    3 = Mildly ill         6 = Severely ill
2 = Borderline mentally ill   4 = Moderately ill     7 = Among the most
                              5 = Markedly ill          extremely ill

# Clinical Global Improvement Scale

Compared to the patient's condition at the beginning of treatment, how much has he/she changed? Circle one (most appropriate).

1 = Very much improved   3 = Minimally improved   6 = Much worse
2 = Much improved        4 = No change            7 = Very much worse
                         5 = Minimally worse

*Source:* National Institute of Mental Health (public domain).

# Children's Yale–Brown Obsessive Compulsive Scale (CY-BOCS)

## GENERAL INSTRUCTIONS

### Overview

This scale is designed to rate the severity of obsessive and compulsive symptoms in children and adolescents, ages 6 to 17 years. It can be administered by a clinician or trained interviewer in a semi-structured fashion. In general, the ratings depend on the child's and parent's report; however, the final rating is based on the clinical judgment of the interviewer. Rate the characteristics of each item over the prior week up until, and including, the time of the interview. Scores should reflect the average of each item for the entire week, unless otherwise specified.

### Informants

Information should be obtained by interviewing the parent(s) (or guardian) and the child together. Sometimes, however, it may also be useful to interview the child or parent alone. Interviewing strategy may vary depending on the age and developmental level of the child or adolescent. All information should be combined to estimate the score for each item. Whenever the CY-BOCS is administered more than once to the same child, as in a medication trial, consistent reporting can be ensured by having the same informant(s) present at each rating session.

Developed by Wayne K. Goodman, MD, Lawrence H. Price, MD, Steven A. Rasmussen, MD, Mark A. Riddle, MD, Judith L. Rapoport, MD, of the Department of Psychiatry and The Child Study Center, Yale University School of Medi.cine; Department of Psychiatry, Brown University School of Medicine; and Child Psychiatry Branch, National Institute of Mental Health
    Investigators interested in using this rating scale should contact Wayne Goodman, MD, at the Clinical Neuroscience Research Unit, Connecticut Mental Health Center, 34 Park Street, New Haven, CT 06508 or Mark Riddle, MD, at the Yale Child Study Center, P.O. Box 3333, New Haven, CT 06510.

Definitions

Before proceeding with the questions, define "obsessions" and "compulsions" for the child and primary caretaker as follows (sometimes, particularly with younger children, the interviewer may prefer using the terms "worries" and "habits"):

> "*Obsessions* are thoughts, ideas, or pictures that keep coming into your mind even though you do not want them to. They may be unpleasant, silly or embarrassing."

> "An *example of an obsession* is the repeated thought that germs or dirt are harming you or other people, or that something unpleasant might happen to you or someone in your family or someone special to you. These are thoughts that keep coming back, over and over again."

> "*Compulsions* are things that you feel you have to do although you may know that they do not make sense. Sometimes you may try to stop from doing them but this might not be possible. You might feel worried or angry or frustrated until you have finished what you have to do."

> "An *example of a compulsion* is the need to wash your hands over and over again even though they are not really dirty, or the need to count up to a certain number while you do certain things."

> "Do you have any questions about what these words called obsessions and compulsions mean?"

Symptom Specificity and Continuity

In some cases, it may be difficult to delineate obsessions and compulsions from other closely related symptoms such as phobias, anxious worries, depressive ruminations, or complex tics. Separate assessment of these symptoms may be necessary. Although potentially difficult, the delineation of obsessions and compulsions from these closely related symptoms is an essential task of the interviewer. (A full discussion of how to make this determination is beyond the scope and purpose of this introduction.) Items marked with an asterix are items where this delineation may be especially troublesome.

Once the interviewer has decided whether or not a particular symptom will be included as an obsession or compulsion on the checklist, every effort should be made to maintain consistency in subsequent rating(s). In a study with multiple ratings over time, it may be useful to review the initial Target

Symptom List (see below) at the beginning of subsequent ratings (prior severity scores should not be reviewed).

## Procedure

*Symptom Checklist.* After reviewing with the child and parent(s) the definitions of obsessions and compulsions, the interview should proceed with a detailed inquiry about the child's symptoms using the Compulsions Checklist and Obsessions Checklist as guides. It may not be necessary to ask about each and every item on the checklist, but each symptom area should be covered to ensure that symptoms are not missed. For most children and adolescents, it is usually easier to begin with compulsions (pages 227 and 228).

*Target Symptom List.* After the Compulsions Checklist is complete, list the four most severe compulsions on the Target Symptom List on page 228. Repeat this process, listing the most severe obsessions on the Target Symptom List on page 224.

*Severity Rating.* After completing the Checklist and Target Symptom List for compulsions, inquire about the severity items: Time Spent, Distress, Resistance, Interference, and Degree of Control (questions 6 through 10 on pages 229 through 232). There are examples of probe questions for each item. Ratings for these items should reflect the interviewer's best estimate from all available information from the past week, with special emphasis on the Target Symptoms. Repeat the above procedure for obsessions (pages 222 through 226). Finally, inquire about and rate questions 11 through 19 on pages 232 through 236. Scores can be recorded on the scoring sheet on pages 237 and 238. *All ratings should be in whole integers.*

## Scoring

All 19 items are rated, but only items 1–10 are used to determine the total score. The total CY-BOCS score is the sum of items 1–10; the obsession and compulsion subtotals are the sums of items 1–5 and 6–10, respectively. At this time, items 1A and 6A are not being used in the scoring.

Items 17 (global severity) and 18 (global improvement) are adapted from the Clinical Global Impression Scale (Guy, 1976) to provide measures of overall functional impairment associated with the presence of obsessive–compulsive symptoms.

Name _____ Date _____

## CY-BOCS OBSESSIONS CHECKLIST

Check all symptoms that apply. (Items marked "*" may or may not be OCD phenomena.)

*Current    Past*

*Contamination Obsessions*

_____   __✔__  Concern with dirt, germs, certain illnesses (e.g., AIDS)

_____   _____  Concerns or disgust with bodily waste or secretions (e.g., urine, feces, saliva)

_____   _____  Excessive concern with enviromental contaminants (e.g., asbestos, radiation, toxic waste)

_____   _____  Excessive concern with household items (e.g., cleaners, solvents)

_____   _____  Excessive concern about animals/insects

_____   _____  Excessively bothered by sticky substances or residues

_____   _____  Concerned will get ill because of contaminant

_____   _____  Concerned will get others ill by spreading contaminant (aggressive)

_____   _____  No concern with consequences of contamination other than how it might feel*

_____   _____  Other (describe): _____

*Aggressive Obsessions*

_____   _____  Fear might harm self

_____   _✔_  Fear might harm others

_✔_   _____  Fear harm will come to self

_____   _✔_  Fear harm will come to others (may be because of something child did or did not do)

_____   _____  Violent or horrific images

_____   _____  Fear of blurting out obscenities or insults

_✔_   _____  Fear of doing something else embarrassing*

_____   _____  Fear will act on unwanted impulses (e.g., to stab a family member)

_____   _____  Fear will steal things

*(cont.)*

✓ _____      Fear will be responsible for something else terrible happening (e.g., fire, burglary, flood)

_____ _____      Other (describe): _____

*Sexual Obsessions*

_____ _____      (Are you having any sexual thoughts? If yes, are they routine or are they repetitive thoughts that you would rather not have or find disturbing? If yes, are they:)

_____ _____      Forbidden or perverse sexual thoughts, images, impulses

_____ _____      Content involves homosexuality*

_____ _____      Sexual behavior towards others (aggressive)

_____ _____      Other (describe): _____

*Hoarding/Saving Obsessions*

_____ _____      Fear of losing things

_____ _____      Other (describe): _____

*Magical Thoughts/Superstitous Obsessions*

_____ _____      Lucky/unlucky numbers, colors, words

_____ _____      Other (describe): _____

*Somatic Obsessions*

✓ _____      Excessive concern with illness or disease*

_____ _____      Excessive concern with body part or aspect of appearance (e.g., dysmorphophobia)*

_____ _____      Other (describe): _____

*Religious Obsessions (Scrupulosity)*

_____ _____      Excessive concern or fear of offending religious objects (God)

_____ _____      Excessive concern with right/wrong, morality

_____ _____      Other (describe): _____

*Miscellaneous Obsessions*

✓ _____      The need to know or remember

✓ _____      Fear of saying certain things

_____ _____      Fear of not saying just the right thing

✓ _____      Intrusive (nonviolent) images

✓ _____      Intrusive sounds, words, music, or numbers

_____ _____      Other (describe): _____

## TARGET SYMPTOM LIST FOR OBSESSIONS

*Obsessions* (Describe, listing by order of severity, with 1 being the most severe, 2 second most severe, etc.):

1. _____

2. _____

3. _____

4. _____


## QUESTIONS ON OBSESSIONS (ITEMS 1–5)

"I am now going to ask you questions about the thoughts you cannot stop thinking about." (Review for the informant(s) the Target Symptoms and refer to them while asking questions 1–5).


### 1. Time Occupied by Obsessive Thoughts

- How much time do you spend thinking about these things?
  (When obsessions occur as brief, intermittent intrusions, it may be impossible to assess time occupied by them in terms of total hours. In such cases, estimate time by determining how frequently they occur. Consider both the number of times the intrusions occur and how many hours of the day are affected).

- How frequently do these thoughts occur?
  (Be sure to exclude ruminations and preccupations which, unlike obsessions, are ego-syntonic and rational [but exaggerated].)

0 – None

1 – Mild       Less than 1 hr/day or occasional intrusion.

2 – Moderate   1 to 3 hrs/day or frequent intrusion.

3 – Severe     Greater than 3 and up to 8 hrs/day or very frequent intrusion.

4 – Extreme    Greater than 8 hrs/day or near constant intrusion.

1B.  Obsession-Free Interval (not included in total score)

  • On the average, what is the longest amount of time each day that you
    are not bothered by the obsessive thoughts?

    0 – None
    1 – Mild        Long symptom-free intervals, more than 8 consecutive
                    hrs/day symptom-free.
    2 – Moderate    Moderately long symptom-free intervals, more than 3
                    and up to 8 consecutive hrs/day symptom-free.
    3 – Severe      Brief symptom-free intervals, from 1 to 3 consecutive
                    hrs/day symptom-free.
    4 – Extreme     Less than 1 consecutive hr/day symptom-free.

2.  Interference due to Obsessive Thoughts

  • How much do these thoughts get in the way of school or doing things
    with friends?

  • Is there anything that you don't do because of them?
    (If currently not in school, determine how much performance would
    be affected if patient were in school.)

    0 – None
    1 – Mild        Slight interference with social or school activities,
                    but overall performance not impaired.
    2 – Moderate    Definite interference with social or school perform-
                    ance, but still manageable.
    3 – Severe      Causes substantial impairment in social or school per-
                    formance.
    4 – Extreme     Incapacitating.

3.  Distress Associated with Obsesssive Thoughts

  • How much do these thoughts bother or upset you?
    (Only rate anxiety/frustration that seems triggered by obsessions, not
    generalized anxiety or anxiety associated with other symptoms.)

    0 – None
    1 – Mild        Infrequent, and not too disturbing.
    2 – Moderate    Frequent, and disturbing, but still manageable.
    3 – Severe      Very frequent, and very disturbing.
    4 – Extreme     Near constant, and disabling distress/frustration.

## 4. Resistance against Obsessions

- How hard do you try to stop the thoughts or ignore them?
  (Only rate effort made to resist, not success or failure in actually controlling the obsessions. How much the patient resists the obsessions may or may not correlate with their ability to control them. Note that this item does not directly measure the severity of the intrusive thoughts; rather it rates a manifestation of health, i.e., the effort the patient makes to counteract the obsessions. Thus, the more the patient tries to resist, the less impaired is this aspect of his functioning. If the obsessions are minimal, the patient may not feel the need to resist them. In such cases, a rating of "0" should be given.)

  0 – None         makes an effort to always resist, or symptoms so minimal doesn't need to actively resist
  1 – Mild         tries to resist most of the time
  2 – Moderate     makes some effort to resist
  3 – Severe       yields to all obsessions without attempting to control them, but does so with some reluctance
  4 – Extreme      completely and willingly yields to all obsessions

## 5. Degree of Control over Obsessive Thoughts

- When you try to fight the thoughts, can you beat them?

- How much control do you have over the thoughts?
  (In contrast to the preceding item on resistance, the ability of the patient to control his obsessions is more closely related to the severity of the intrusive thoughts.)

  0 – Complete control
  1 – Much control        Usually able to stop or divert obsessions with some effort and concentration.
  2 – Moderate control    Sometimes able to stop or divert obsessions.
  3 – Little control      Rarely successful in stopping obsessions, can only divert attention with difficulty.
  4 – No control          Experienced as completely involuntary, rarely able to even momentarily divert thinking.

Name _____ Date _____

## CY-BOCS COMPULSIONS CHECKLIST

Check all symptoms that apply. (Items marked "*" may or may not be OCD phenomena.)

*Current*    *Past*

*Washing/Cleaning Compulsions*

☑ _____ Excessive or ritualized handwashing

_____ _____ Excessive or ritualized showering, bathing, toothbrushing, grooming, toilet routine

☑ _____ Excessive cleaning of items; such as personal clothes or important objects

_____ _____ Other measures to prevent or remove contact with contaminants

_____ _____ Other (describe): _____

*Checking Compulsions*

_____ _____ Checking locks, toys, school books/items, etc.

_____ _____ Checking associated with getting washed, dressed, or undressed

_____ _____ Checking that did not/will not harm others

_____ _____ Checking that did not/will not harm self

_____ _____ Checking that nothing terrible did/will happen

_____ _____ Checking that did not make mistake

_____ _____ Checking tied to somatic obsessions

_____ _____ Other (describe): _____

*Repeating Rituals*

_____ _____ Rereading, erasing, or rewriting

_____ _____ Need to repeat routine activities (e.g., in/out of doorway, up/down from chair)

_____ _____ Other (describe): _____

*Counting Compulsions*

_____ _____ Objects, certain numbers, words, etc.

_____ _____ Describe: _____

*(cont.)*

*Ordering/Arranging*

____   ____   Need for symmetry/evening up (e.g., lining items up a certain way or arranging personal items in specific patterns)

____   ____   Other (describe): _____

*Hoarding/Saving Compulsions*
(distinguish from hobbies and concern with objects of monetary or sentimental value)

____   ____   Difficulty throwing things away, saving bits of paper, string, etc.

____   ____   Other (describe): _____

*Excessive Games/Superstitious Behaviors*
(distinguish from age-appropriate magical games)

____   ____   (e.g., array of behavior, such as stepping over certain spots on a floor, touching an object/self certain number of times as a routine game to avoid something bad from happening.)

____   ____   Other (describe): _____

*Rituals Involving Other Persons*

____   ____   The need to involve another person (usually a parent) in ritual (e.g., asking a parent to repeatedly answer the same question, making mother perform certain meal-time rituals involving specific utensils).*

____   ____   Other (describe): _____

*Miscellaneous Compulsions*

____   ____   Mental rituals (other than checking/counting)

____   ____   Need to tell, ask, or confess

____   ____   Measures (not checking) to prevent harm to self ___; harm to others ___; terrible consequences ___

____   ____   Ritualized eating behaviors*

____   ____   Excessive list making*

____   ____   Need to touch, tap, rub*

____   ____   Need to do things (e.g., touch or arrange) until it *feels just right)*

____   ____   Rituals involving blinking or staring*

____   ____   Trichotillomania (hair-pulling)*

____   ____   Other self-damaging or self-mutilating behaviors*

____   ____   Other (describe): _____

## TARGET SYMPTOM LIST FOR COMPULSIONS

*Compulsions* (Describe, listing by order of severity, with 1 being the most severe, 2 second most severe, etc.):

1. _____

2. _____

3. _____

4. _____

## QUESTIONS ON COMPULSIONS (ITEMS 6–10)

"I am now going to ask you questions about the habits you can't stop." (Review for the informant[s] the Target Symptoms and refer to them while asking questions 6–10).

6A. Time Spent Performing Compulsive Behaviors

- How much time do you spend doing these things?

- How much longer than most people does it take to complete your usual daily activities because of the habits?
  (When compulsions occur as brief, intermittent behaviors, it may be impossible to assess time spent performing them in terms of total hours. In such cases, estimate time by determining how frequently they are performed. Consider both the number of times compulsions are performed and how many hours of the day are affected).

- How often do you do these habits?
  (In most cases compulsions are observable behaviors [e.g., handwashing], but there are instances in which compulsions are not observable [e.g., silent checking].)

  0 – None
  1 – Mild          Spends less than 1 hr/day performing compulsions, or occasional performance of compulsive behaviors.
  2 – Moderate      Spends from 1 to 3 hrs/day performing compulsions, or frequent performance of compulsive behaviors
  3 – Severe        Spends more than 3 and up to 8 hrs/day performing compulsions, or very frequent performance of compulsions.

4 – Extreme    Spends more than 8 hrs/day performing compulsions, or near constant performance of compulsive behaviors (too numerous to count).

## 6B. Compulsion-Free Interval

- How long can you go without performing compulsive behavior? (If necessary ask: What is the longest block of time in which [your habits] compulsions are absent?)

0 – No symptoms
1 – Mild        Long symptom-free interval, more than 8 consecutive hrs/day symptom-free.
2 – Moderate    Moderately long symptom-free interval, more than 3 and up to 8 consecutive hrs/day symptom-free.
3 – Severe      Short symptom-free interval, from 1 to 3 consecutive hrs/day symptom-free.
4 – Extreme     Less than 1 consecutive hr/day symptom-free.

## 7. Interference due to Compulsive Behaviors

- How much do these habits get in the way of school or doing things with friends?

- Is there anything you don't do because of them? (If currently not in school, determine how much performance would be affected if patient were in school.)

0 – None
1 – Mild        Slight interference with social or school activities, but overall performance not impaired.
2 – Moderate    Definite interference with social or school performance, but still manageable.
3 – Severe      Causes substantial impairment in social or school performance.
4 – Extreme     Incapacitating.

## 8. Distress Associated with Compulsive Behavior

- How would you feel if prevented from carrying out your habits?

- How upset would you become?
  (Rate degree of distress/frustration patient would experience if per-

formance of the compulsion were suddenly interrupted without reassurance being offered. In most, but not all cases, performing compulsions reduces anxiety/frustration.

- How upset do you get while carrying out your habits until you feel satisfied?

0 – None

1 – Mild  Only slightly anxious/frustrated if compulsions prevented, or only slight anxiety/frustration during performance of compulsions.

2 – Moderate Reports that anxiety/frustration would mount but remain manageable if compulsions prevented. Anxiety/frustration increases but remains manageable during performance of compulsions.

3 – Severe  Prominent and very disturbing increase in anxiety/frustration if compulsions interrupted. Prominent and very disturbing increase in anxiety/frustration during performance of compulsions.

4 – Extreme  Incapacitating anxiety/frustration from any intervention aimed at modifying activity. Incapacitating anxiety/frustration develops during performance of compulsions.

## 9. Resistance against Compulsions

- How much do you try to fight the habits?
(Only rate effort made to resist, not success or failure in actually controlling the compulsions. How much the patient resists the compulsions may or may not correlate with his ability to control them. Note that this item does not directly measure the severity of the compulsions; rather it rates a manifestation of health, i.e., the effort the patient makes to counteract the compulsions. Thus, the more the patient tries to resist, the less impaired is this aspect of his functioning. If the compulsions are minimal, the patient may not feel the need to resist them. In such cases, a rating of "0" should be given.)

0 – None  Makes an effort to always resist, or symptoms so minimal doesn't need to actively resist.

1 – Mild  Tries to resist most of the time.

2 – Moderate Makes some effort to resist.

3 – Severe     Yields to almost all compulsions without attempting
               to control them, but does so with some reluctance.
4 – Extreme    Completely and willingly yields to all compulsions.

## 10. Degree of Control over Compulsive Behavior

- How strong is the feeling that you have to carry out the habit(s)?

- When you try to fight them, what happens?

(For the advanced child, ask:)

- How much control do you have over the habits?
  (In contrast to the preceding item on resistance, the ability of the
  patient to control his compulsions is more closely related to the
  severity of the compulsions.)

0 – Complete control
1 – Much control         Experiences pressure to perform the beha-
                         vior, but usually able to exercise voluntary
                         control over it.
2 – Moderate control     Moderate control, strong pressure to perform
                         behavior, can control it only with difficulty.
3 – Little control       Little control, very strong drive to perform
                         behavior, must be carried to completion,
                         can only delay with difficulty.
4 – No control           No control, drive to perform behavior ex-
                         perienced as completely involuntary and
                         overpowering, rarely able to delay activity
                         (even momentarily).

## 11. Insight into Obsessions and Compulsions

- Do you think your concern or behaviors are reasonable? (Pause)

- What do you think would happen if you did not perform the compul-
  sion(s)?

- Are you convinced something would really happen?
  (Rate patient's insight into the senselessness or excessiveness of his
  obsession(s) and compulsion(s) based on beliefs expressed at the time
  of the interview.)

0 – None        Excellent insight, fully rational.

1 – Mild          Good insight, readily acknowledges absurdity or ex-
                  cessiveness of thoughts or behaviors but does not
                  seem completely convinced that there isn't some-
                  thing besides anxiety to be concerned about (i.e.,
                  has lingering doubts).

2 – Moderate      Fair insight, reluctantly admits thoughts or behavior
                  seem unreasonable or excessive, but wavers. May
                  have some unrealistic fears, but no fixed convic-
                  tions.

3 – Severe        Poor insight, maintains that thoughts or behaviors
                  are not reasonable or excessive, but wavers. May
                  have some unrealistic fears, but acknowledges valid-
                  ity of contrary evidence (i.e., overvalued ideas pre-
                  sent).

4 – Extreme       Lacks insight, delusional, definitely convinced that
                  concerns and behavior are reasonable, unresponsive
                  to contrary evidence.

## 12. Avoidance

- Have you been avoiding doing anything, going any place, or being with anyone because of your obsessional thoughts or out of concern you will perform compulsions?

(If yes, then ask:)

- How much do you avoid? (Note what is avoided on symptom list.) (Rate degree to which patient deliberately tries to avoid things. Sometimes compulsions are designed to "avoid" contact with something that the patient fears. For example, excessive washing of fruits and vegetables to remove "germs" would be designated as a compulsion not as an avoidant behavior. If the patient stopped eating fruits and vegetables, then this would constitute avoidance).

0 – None

1 – Mild          Minimal avoidance.

2 – Moderate      Some avoidance; clearly present.

3 – Severe        Much avoidance; avoidance prominent.

4 – Extreme       Very extensive avoidance; patient does almost every-
                  thing he/she can to avoid triggering symptoms.

13. Degree of Indecisiveness

- Do you have trouble making decisions about little things that other people might not think twice about (e.g., which clothes to put on in the morning; which brand of cereal to buy)?
(Exclude difficulty making decisions which reflect ruminative thinking. Ambivalence concerning rationally based difficult choices should also be excluded.)

0 – None
1 – Mild          Some trouble making decisions about minor things.
2 – Moderate      Freely reports significant trouble making decisions that others would not think twice about.
3 – Severe        Continual weighing of pros and cons about nonessentials.
4 – Extreme       Unable to make any decisions, disabling.

14. Overvalued Sense of Responsibility

- Do you feel overly responsible for what you do and for the effects of your actions?

- Do you blame yourself for things that are not within your control?
(Distinguish from normal feelings of responsibility, feelings of worthlessness, and pathological guilt. A guilt-ridden person experiences himself or his actions as bad or evil.)

0 – None
1 – Mild          Only mentioned on questioning, slight sense of over-responsibility.
2 – Moderate      Ideas stated spontaneously, clearly present; patient experiences significant sense of overresponsibility for events outside his/her reasonable control.
3 – Severe        Ideas prominent and pervasive; deeply concerned he/she is responsible for events clearly outside his control, self-blaming farfetched and nearly irrational.
4 – Extreme       Delusional sense of responsibility (e.g., if an earthquake occurs 3,000 miles away patient blames himself because he didn't perform his compulsion).

15. Pervasive Slowness/Disturbance of Inertia

- Do you have difficulty starting or finishing tasks?

- Do many routine activities take longer than they should?

(Distinguish from psychomotor retardation secondary to depression. Rate increased time spent performing routine activities even when specific obsessions cannot be identified).

0 – None

1 – Mild         Occasional delay in starting or finishing tasks/activities.

2 – Moderate   Frequent prolongation of routine activities but tasks usually completed, frequently late.

3 – Severe     Pervasive and marked difficulty initiating and completing routine tasks, usually late.

4 – Extreme    Unable to start or complete routine tasks without full assistance.

## 16. Pathological Doubting

- After you complete an activity do you doubt whether you performed it correctly?

- Do you doubt whether you did it at all?

- When carrying out routine activities do you find that you don't trust your senses (i.e., what you see, hear, or touch)?

0 – None

1 – Mild         Only mentioned on questioning, slight pathological doubt, examples given may be within normal range.

2 – Moderate   Ideas stated spontaneously, clearly present and apparent in some of patient's behaviors; patient bothered by significant pathological doubt. Some effect on performance but still manageable.

3 – Severe     Uncertainty about perceptions or memory prominent; pathological doubt frequently effects performance.

4 – Extreme    Uncertainty about perceptions constantly present; pathological doubt substantially effects almost all activities, incapacitating (e.g., patient states "my mind doesn't trust what my eyes see").

## 17. Global Severity

Interviewer's judgment of the overall severity of the patient's illness. Rated from 0 (no illness) to 6 (most severe patient seen).

(Consider the degree of distress reported by the patient, the symptoms observed, and the functional impairment reported. Your judgment is required both in averaging this data as well as weighing the reliability or accuracy of the data obtained.)

| | |
|---|---|
| 0 – No illness | |
| 1 – Slight | Illness slight, doubtful, transient; no functional impairment. |
| 2 – Mild | Little functional impairment. |
| 3 – Moderate | Functions with effort. |
| 4 – Moderate–severe | Limited functioning. |
| 5 – Severe | Functions mainly with assistance. |
| 6 – Extremely severe | Completely nonfunctional. |

## 18. Global Improvement

Rate total overall improvement present *since the initial rating* whether or not, in your judgment, it is due to treatment.

0 – Very much worse
1 – Much worse
2 – Minimally worse
3 – No change
4 – Minimally improved
5 – Much improved
6 – Very much improved

## 19. Reliability

Rate the overall reliability of the rating scores obtained. Factors that may affect reliability include the patient's cooperativeness and his/her natural ability to communicate. The type and severity of obsessive–compulsive symptoms present may interfere with the patient's concentration, attention, or freedom to speak spontaneously (e.g., the content of some obsessions may cause the patient to choose his words very carefully).

| | |
|---|---|
| 0 – Excellent | No reason to suspect data unreliable. |
| 1 – Good | Factor(s) present that may adversely affect reliability. |
| 2 – Fair | Factor(s) present that definitely reduce reliability. |
| 3 – Poor | Very low reliability. |

## CHILDREN'S YALE–BROWN OBSESSIVE COMPULSIVE SCALE

CY-BOCS total (add items 1–10) ___

Patient name _____ Date _____

Patient ID _____ Rater _____

| | None | Mild | Moderate | Severe | Extreme |
|---|---|---|---|---|---|
| 1. Time spent on obsessions | 0 | 1 | 2 | 3 | 4 |

| | No symptoms | Long | Moderately long | Short | Extremely short |
|---|---|---|---|---|---|
| 1b. Obsession-free interval (do not add to subtotal or total score) | 0 | 1 | 2 | 3 | 4 |

| | | | | | |
|---|---|---|---|---|---|
| 2. Interference from obsessions | 0 | 1 | 2 | 3 | 4 |
| 3. Distress of obsessions | 0 | 1 | 2 | 3 | 4 |

| | Always resists | | | | Completely yields |
|---|---|---|---|---|---|
| 4. Resistance | 0 | 1 | 2 | 3 | 4 |

| | Complete control | Much control | Moderate control | Little control | No control |
|---|---|---|---|---|---|
| 5. Control over obsessions | 0 | 1 | 2 | 3 | 4 |

*Obsession subtotal (add items 1–5)* ___

| | None | Mild | Moderate | Severe | Extreme |
|---|---|---|---|---|---|
| 6. Time spent on compulsions | 0 | 1 | 2 | 3 | 4 |

| | No symptoms | Long | Moderately long | Short | Extremely short |
|---|---|---|---|---|---|
| 6b. Compulsion-free interval (do not add to subtotal or total score) | 0 | 1 | 2 | 3 | 4 |

| | | | | | |
|---|---|---|---|---|---|
| 7. Interference from compulsions | 0 | 1 | 2 | 3 | 4 |
| 8. Distress from compulsions | 0 | 1 | 2 | 3 | 4 |

|                         | Always<br>resists |   |   |   | Completely<br>yields |
| ----------------------- | :---: | :---: | :---: | :---: | :---: |
| 9. Resistance           | 0     | 1     | 2     | 3     | 4     |

|                         | Complete<br>control | Much<br>control | Moderate<br>control | Little<br>control | No<br>control |
| ----------------------- | :---: | :---: | :---: | :---: | :---: |
| 10. Control over<br>compulsions | 0 | 1 | 2 | 3 | 4 |

*Compulsion subtotal (add items 6–10)* ___

|                         | Excellent |   |   |   | Absent |
| ----------------------- | :---: | :---: | :---: | :---: | :---: |
| 11. Insight into<br>O-C symptoms | 0 | 1 | 2 | 3 | 4 |

|                               | None | Mild | Moderate | Severe | Extreme |
| ----------------------------- | :---: | :---: | :---: | :---: | :---: |
| 12. Avoidance                 | 0 | 1 | 2 | 3 | 4 |
| 13. Indecisiveness            | 0 | 1 | 2 | 3 | 4 |
| 14. Pathologic responsibility | 0 | 1 | 2 | 3 | 4 |
| 15. Slowness                  | 0 | 1 | 2 | 3 | 4 |
| 16. Pathologic doubting       | 0 | 1 | 2 | 3 | 4 |

| 17. Global severity    | 0 | 1 | 2 | 3 | 4 | 5 | 6 |
| ---------------------- | :---: | :---: | :---: | :---: | :---: | :---: | :---: |
| 18. Global improvement | 0 | 1 | 2 | 3 | 4 | 5 | 6 |

| 19. Reliability | Excellent = 0   Good = 1   Fair = 2   Poor = 3 |
| --------------- | ---------------------------------------------- |

# Leyton Obsessional Inventory

Your name: _____ Date: _____

*Instructions:* Please place a check in the appropriate box for each question.

If answer is yes:

   0—This habit does not stop me from doing other things I want to do.

   1—This stops me a little or wastes a little of my time.

   2—This stops me from doing other things or wastes some of my time.

   3—This stops me from doing a lot of things and wastes a lot of my time.

| | No | Yes | | |
|---|---|---|---|---|
| | | 0 | 1 | 2 | 3 |
| 1. Do you often feel like you have to do certain things even though you know you don't really have to? | | | | |
| 2. Do thoughts or words ever keep going over and over in your mind? | | | | |
| 3. Do you have to check things several times? | | | | |
| 4. Do you hate dirt and dirty things? | | | | |
| 5. Do you ever feel that if something has been used or touched by someone else it is spoiled for you? | | | | |
| 6. Do you ever worry about being clean enough? | | | | |
| 7. Are you fussy about keeping your hands clean? | | | | |
| 8. When you put things away at night, do they have to be put away just right? | | | | |

*(cont.)*

9. Do you get angry if other students mess up your desk?

10. Do you spend a lot of extra time checking your homework to make sure it is just right?

11. Do you ever have to do things over and over a certain number of times before they seem quite right?

12. Do you ever have to count several times or go through numbers in your head?

13. Do you ever have trouble finishing your school work or chores because you have to do something over and over again?

14. Do you have a favorite or special number that you like to count up to a lot or do things just that number of times?

15. Do you often have a bad conscience because you've done something even though no one else thinks it's bad?

16. Do you worry a lot if you've done something not exactly the way you like?

17. Do you have trouble making up your mind?

18. Do you go over things a lot that you have done because you aren't sure that they were the right things to do?

19. Do you move or talk in just a special way to avoid bad luck?

20. Do you have special numbers or words you say, just because it keeps bad luck away or bad things away?

Appendix III

# Resources, Tips for Parents, and Guidelines

## Resources

Support groups are an invaluable part of treatment. These groups provide a forum for mutual acceptance, understanding, and self-discovery. Participants develop a sense of camaraderie with other attendees because they have all lived with OCD. People new to OCD can talk to others who have learned successful strategies for coping with the illness.

### ORGANIZATIONS

The Obsessive–Compulsive Foundation
P.O. Box 70
Milford, CT
203-878-5669

Premier lay and professional advocacy organization for persons of all ages with OCD and their family members.

You also may wish to point your web browser at the OC Foundation's web site: **http:/pages.prodigy.com/alwillen/ocf.html,** where you'll find a listing of other OCD resources on the web, as well as lots of useful information regarding OCD in children, adolescents, and adults.

The Obsessive–Compulsive Information Center
2711 Allen Boulevard
Middleton, WI 53562
608-836-7000

The OCIC, which is staffed by medical librarians, provides access to the published literature on OCD and publishes very useful guides about OCD and some OC spectrum disorders, such as trichotillomania, in children and adults.

The Anxiety Disorders Association of America
6000 Executive Avenue, Suite 513
Rockville, MD 20852
301-231-9350

The Anxiety Disorders Association of America provides a central clearinghouse for patients with, and professionals interested in, the diagnosis and treatment of all anxiety disorders, including but not limited to OCD.

The Tourette Syndrome Association
42-40 Bell Boulevard
Bayside, NY 11361-2874
718-224-2999

The Tourette Syndrome Association provides a central clearinghouse for patients with, and professionals interested in, the diagnosis and treatment of the tic disorders. Because tic disorders often overlap with OCD, the TSA includes a wealth of information about the overlap between these two conditions.

## PUBLICATIONS ABOUT OCD

For more information about OCD, we recommend:

Baer, L. (1991). *Getting control.* Boston, MA: Little, Brown.
Ciarrocchi, J. (1995). *The doubting disease.* Mawhah, NJ: Paulist Press.

Foa, E. B., & Wilson, R. (1991). *Stop obsessing!* New York: Bantam.

Francis, G., & Gragg, R. (1996). *Childhood obsessive compulsive disorder.* Thousand Oaks, CA: Sage.

Fruehling, J. (1997). *Drug treatment of OCD in children and adolescents.* Milford, CT: OC Foundation.

Greist, J. (1994). *Obsessive compulsive disorder: A guide* (2nd ed.). Madison, WI: Obsessive Compulsive Information Center.

Greist, J., Jefferson, J., & Marks, I. (1989). *Anxiety and its treatment.* New York: Bantam.

Johnston, H. (1993). *Obsessive compulsive disorder in children and adolescents.* Madison, WI: Child Psychopharmacology Information Center.

March, J. S. (Ed.). (1995). *Anxiety disorders in children and adolescents.* New York: Guilford Press.

Neziroglu, F., & Yaryura-Tobias, J. (1991). *Over and over again: Understanding obsessive compulsive disorder.* Lexington, MA: Lexington Books.

Rapoport, J. (1989). *The boy who couldn't stop washing.* New York: Dutton.

Schwartz, J. (1996). *Brain lock.* New York: HarperCollins.

Steketee, G. S., & White, K. (1990). *When once is not enough: Help for obsessive-compulsives.* Oakland, CA: Harbinger.

van Noppen, B., Pato, M., & Rasmussen, S. (1993). *Learning to live with obsessive compulsive disorder* (2nd ed.). Milford, CT: OC Foundation.

## PUBLICATIONS ABOUT OTHER CONDITIONS

Depending on need, we also recommend the following materials that address the more common comorbid conditions that complicate the treatment of pediatric OCD:

Barkley, R. A. (1997). *Defiant children* (2nd ed.): *A clinician's manual for parent training.* New York: Guilford Press.
  • A straightforward manual to guide treatment of the child with a DRP on a session-by-session basis. Includes rating scales and parent handouts.

Barlow, D. H. (1992). Cognitive-behavioral approaches to panic disorder and social phobia. *Bulletin of the Menninger Clinic, 56*(2, Suppl A), A14–A28.

Barlow, D. H., & Craske, M. (1989). *Mastery of your anxiety and panic.* Albany, NY: Graywind.
  • An elegant approach to the treatment of social phobia and panic disorder in adults; can easily be downsized to be made age appropriate for children and adolescents.

Conners, C., Wells, K., March, J. S., & Fiore, C. (1994). Methodological issues in the multimodal treatment of the disruptive behavior disorders. In L. Greenhill (Ed.), *Psychiatric clinics of North America: Disruptive behavior disorders* (pp. 361–378). Philadelphia: Saunders.

Deblinger, E., McLeer, S. V., & Henry, D. (1990). Cognitive behavioral treatment for sexually abused children suffering post-traumatic stress: preliminary findings. *Journal of the American Academy of Child and Adolescent Psychiatry, 29*(5), 747–752.

Dornbush, M., & Pruit, S. (1995). *Teaching the tiger: A handbook for individuals involved in the education of students with attention deficit disorders, Tourette syndrome or obsessive–compulsive disorder.* Duarte, CA: Hope Press.
  • The absolute best step-by-step survival guide to navigating through schools. Includes very helpful suggestions for school staff working with a child with OCD. Also covers social needs, learning style differences, and your legal rights.

Erhardt, D., & Baker, B. L. (1990). The effects of behavioral parent training on families with young hyperactive children. *Journal of Behavior Therapy and Experimental Psychiatry, 21*(2), 121–132.

Foa, E. B., & Kozak, M. (1985). Emotional processing of fear: Exposure to corrective information. *Psychological Bulletin, 90,* 20–35.

Foa, E. B., & Rothbaum, E. (1992). Cognitive-behavioral treatment of posttraumatic stress disorder. In P. Saigh (Ed.), *Post-traumatic stress disorder: A behavioral approach to diagnosis and treatment* (pp. 85–110). Needham Heights, MA: Allyn and Bacon.

Foa, E. B., Steketee, G. S., & Rothbaum, B. (1989). Behavioral/cognitive conceptualizations of post-traumatic stress disorder. *Behavior Therapy, 20,* 155–176.

Forehand, R. L., & McMahon, R. J. (1981). *Helping the noncompliant child: A clinician's guide to parent training.* New York: Guilford Press.
  • Another excellent guide to helping manage oppositional behavior.

Francis, G., & Beidel, D. (1995). Cognitive behavioral psychotherapy. In J. S. March (Ed.), *Anxiety disorders in children and adolescents* (pp. 321–340). New York: Guilford Press.
  • An excellent introduction to CBT for youth with anxiety disorders. Each treatment chapter presents a detailed discussion of CBT. The treatment section includes a discussion of how to set up a multidisciplinary anxiety disorders clinic.

Heimberg, R. G., & Juster, H. R. (1994). Treatment of social phobia in cognitive-behavioral groups. *Journal of Clinical Psychiatry, 55*(Suppl. 6), 38–46.

Hibbs, E., & Jensen, P. (Eds.). (1996). *Psychosocial treatments for child and adolescent disorders: Empirically based approaches.* Washington, DC: American Psychological Press.

- Marvelous and current descriptions of empirically supported to treatment for all the major clusters of child and adolescent psychopathology written by the experts who developed those treatments.

Horn, W., Ialongo, N., Pascoe, J., Grenberg, G., Packard, T., Lopez, M., Wagner, A., & Puttler, L. (1991). Additive effects of psychostimulants, parent training, and self-control therapy with ADHD children. *Journal of the American Academy of Child and Adolescent Psychiatry, 30,* 233–240.

Kendall, P. C. (1991). *Child and adolescent therapy: Cognitive-behavioral procedures.* New York: Guilford Press.
- A seminal text on cognitive-behavioral therapy covering a range of child and adolescent disorders.

Kendall, P. C. (1993). Cognitive-behavioral therapies with youth: Guiding theory, current status, and emerging developments. *Journal of Consulting and Clinical Psychology, 61*(2), 235–247.

Kendall, P. C., Kortlander, E., Chansky, T. E., & Brady, E. U. (1992). Comorbidity of anxiety and depression in youth: Treatment implications. Special section: Comorbidity and treatment implications. *Journal of Consulting and Clinical Psychology, 60*(6), 869–880.

Kendall, P. C., & Panichelli-Mindel, S. M. (1995). Cognitive-behavioral treatments. *Journal of Abnormal Child Psychology, 23*(1), 107–124.

Lewinsohn, P. M., Clarke, G. N., & Rohde, P. (1994). *Psychological approaches to the treatment of depression in adolescents.* New York: Plenum.
- An introduction to CBT for depression by the folks who do it best.

Lochman, J., Lampron, L., Gemmer, T., & Harris, S. (1987). Anger coping intervention with aggressive children: A guide to implementation in school settings. In P. Keller & S. Heyman (Eds.), *Innovations In clinical practice: A source book* (Vol. 6, pp. 339–356). Sarasota, FL: Professional Resource Exchange.
- Widely used in prevention intervention programs, anger coping is a useful modality to incorporate into treatment protocols for DRBs, depression, and anxiety (i.e., wherever children have difficulty with bossy tempers).

March, J. S., & Mulle, K. (1995). Manualized cognitive-behavioral psychotherapy for obsessive-compulsive disorder in childhood: A preliminary single case study. *Journal of Anxiety Disorders, 9*(2), 175–184.

March, J. S., Mulle, K., & Herbel, B. (1994). Behavioral psychotherapy for children and adolescents with obsessive-compulsive disorder: An open trial of a new protocol driven treatment package. *Journal of the American Academy of Child and Adolescent Psychiatry, 33*(3), 333–341.

March, J. S., Wells, K., & Conners, C. (1995). Attention-deficit/hyperactivity disorder: Part I. Diagnosis. *Journal of Practical Psychiatry and Behavioral Health, 1*(4), 219–223.

March, J. S., Wells, K., & Conners, C. (1996). Attention-deficit/hyperactivity disorder: Part II. Treatment. *Journal of Practical Psychiatry and Behavioral Health, 2*(1), 23–32.
• A detailed summary of the diagnosis and treatment of ADHD.

Marks, I. M., Lelliott, P., Basoglu, M., Noshirvani, H., Monteiro, W., Cohen, D., & Kasvikis, Y. (1988). Clomipramine, self-exposure and therapist-aided exposure for obsessive-compulsive rituals. *British Journal of Psychiatry, 152*(522), 522–534.

Moreau, D., Mufson, L., Weissman, M. M., & Klerman, G. L. (1991). Interpersonal psychotherapy for adolescent depression: Description of modification and preliminary application. *Journal of the American Academy of Child and Adolescent Psychiatry, 30*(4), 642–651.

Mufson, L., Moreau, D., Weissman, M. M., & Klerman, G. L. (1993). *Interpersonal psychotherapy for depressed adolescents.* New York: Guilford Press.
• Another excellent approach to the depressed youngster, especially when relationship and/or grief issues are paramount.

Mufson, L., Moreau, D., Weissman, M. M., & Wickramaratne, P. (1994). Modification of interpersonal psychotherapy with depressed adolescents (IPT-A): Phase I and II studies. *Journal of the American Academy of Child and Adolescent Psychiatry, 33*(5), 695–705.

Pennington, B. F. (1991). *Diagnosing learning disorders: A neuropsychological framework.* New York: Guilford Press.
• An excellent introduction to the overlap of LD and psychopathology, this book also serves as an introduction to an LD model developmental psychopathology.

Pfiffner, L., & Barkley, R. A. (1990). Educational placement and classroom management. In R. A. Barkley, *Attention-deficit hyperactivity disorder: A handbook for diagnosis and treatment* (pp. 498–539). New York: Guilford Press.

Thyer, B. A. (1991). Diagnosis and treatment of child and adolescent anxiety disorders. *Behavior Modification, 15*(3), 310–325.

van Oppen, P., de Haan, e., van Balkan, A., Spinhoven, P., Hoodguin, K., & van Dyck, R. (1995). Cognitive therapy and exposure in vivo in the treatment of obsessive compulsive disorder. *Behaviour Research and Therapy, 33*(4), 370–390.

Vitulano, L. A., King, R. A., Scahill, L., & Cohen, D. J. (1992). Behavioral treatment of children and adolescents with trichotillomania. *Journal of the American Academy of Child and Adolescent Psychiatry, 31*(1), 139–146.

Wells, K. (1995). Family therapy. In J. S. March (Ed.), *Anxiety disorders in children and adolescents* (pp. 401–419). New York: Guilford Press.
• An excellent discussion of how to work with anxious children from the family therapy perspective

# Tips for Parents

You and your child are about to embark on a time-limited treatment program for children and adolescents with OCD developed in the Program for Child and Adolescent Anxiety Disorders at Duke University. This treatment package, which in research studies has shown itself to be an effective treatment for OCD in young persons, has been used by thousands of clinicians around the world to help children and adolescents do away with OCD.

Your child's treatment will consist of 12–20 sessions of cognitive-behavioral psychotherapy (CBT). The BT in CBT stands for behavior therapy. Behavior therapy means that you can change your thoughts and feelings by first changing your behavior. In OCD, behavior therapy means exposing oneself to feared situations (exposure) and refraining from performing rituals (response prevention). Cognitive therapy (CT), which is usually added to exposure and response prevention (E/RP), addresses the catastrophic thinking and exaggerated sense of personal responsibility commonly seen in patients with OCD. Thus, behavior therapy (the BT in CBT) more properly refers to E/RP, while CT + E/RP is termed CBT.

As the name suggests, obsessive–compulsive disorder (OCD) is characterized by both obsessions and compulsions. Obsessions are unwanted, persistent thoughts, images, or urges that are accompanied by unpleasant feelings such as anxiety, disgust, or guilt. Common examples include contamination/germ fears, fear of harming self or others, aggressive or sexual thoughts, and "just so" worries. "Just so" OCD usually involves a felt need for exactness or symmetry rather than an idea about perfectionism. Compulsions, which are sometimes termed rituals, are acts that are performed to reduce the uncomfortable feelings, thoughts, and urges involved in obsessions. Compulsions, which include cleaning, washing, checking, ordering/arranging, counting, repeating, and hoarding or collecting, are usually performed in a rule-bound manner and are often bizarre. For example, an 8-year-old boy with "just so" OCD and counting rituals may have to trace and retrace his letters eight times or more, making it hard from him to complete his school work.

OCD in children and adolescents is more common than was once thought. Between 1 in 100 and 1 in 200 young persons is affected at any given time. This means that there are 3 or 4 youngsters with OCD in the average-size elementary school and up to 20 in a large urban high school. Since most of us don't know that many children with OCD, researchers believe that a large number must be suffering in silence. Although there is a great deal of overlap between boys and girls with OCD, research has also shown that OCD on average looks a bit different in boys and girls. Boys have more "just so" feelings, and are more likely to have tics and attention-deficit/hyperactivity disorder (ADHD). Boys' OCD symptoms are more likely to begin during the elementary school years. Girls exhibit more fears and anxiety, are more likely to be depressed, and their OCD symptoms are more likely to start during early adolescence.

While OCD in children looks like OCD in adults, and responds to both behavioral psychotherapy and to specific anti-OCD medications, OCD in kids poses a unique treatment challenge because young persons: (1) typically have more trouble seeing obsessions as senseless and compulsions as excessive, especially in the middle of an attack of OCD; (2) tend to be embarrassed by their obsessions and compulsions, and so try to keep them secret; (3) not uncommonly have more difficulty tolerating anxiety; and (4) more frequently involve family members in rituals. Thus, the treatment program we have devised includes strategies for sharpening insight, managing anxiety, and working with families, along with the techniques—mainly exposure and response prevention (E/RP)—necessary to eliminate OCD symptoms. During these sessions, you and your child will receive information about OCD, instructions about how to "boss back" OCD, and a "tool kit" for coping with anxiety, and will have an opportunity to practice these strategies with the therapist. In addition, your child will choose a series of homework assignments that help him or her "boss back" OCD.

Parents often ask, "How can we help?" First, the program includes two parent sessions. In addition, we prepared the following instruction sheets (coaching tips) to help explain particular elements of the treatment program. These parent coaching tips offer practical information and suggestions on how you can best participate in your child's treatment process.

## SETTING THE STAGE FOR TREATMENT

### Tip 1. What Is OCD?

While experts still aren't sure about how OCD gets started, most agree that OCD is a neurobehavioral disorder, that is, a brain and behavior problem that affects a child's thoughts, feelings, and behaviors in a very specific fashion. As a neurobehavioral illness, OCD cannot, in any way, be viewed as your child's "fault," or as something your child could stop "if he or she just tried harder." Rather, OCD is best viewed as a "short circuit," "hiccup," and/or "volume control" problem in the brain's "worry computer" that your child cannot stop by himself or herself. This "worry computer" inappropriately sends fear cues that do not deserve such attention. These fear cues are what we call obsessions.

## Tip 2. What Are Obsessions?

Obsessions are unwanted thoughts, urges, or images that are accompanied by negative feelings. A common obsession is the fear of contaminating oneself or someone else by touching something "germy." Not surprisingly, you can't see obsessions, but you may notice that your child appears distracted or inattentive. When the brain gives these unwanted fear cues, the child's responses show up as ritualized behaviors called compulsions.

## Tip 3. What Are Compulsions?

Compulsions are actions designed to make these thoughts go away and to relieve accompanying anxiety or other bad feelings. For example, excessive handwashing is a common ritual for patients with contamination fears. Avoiding "contamination" is also common, and can produce considerable distress and dysfunction. It is easy to see compulsions as bad behavior rather than as a natural, if self-defeating, response to obsessions. On the other hand, your child almost certainly is frustrated and depressed by his or her inability to resist OCD, and adding to the burdens imposed by OCD isn't helpful. By viewing OCD as a specific brain problem, you and your child can let go of the notion that either you or your child is somehow at fault, thereby taking a first step toward effective treatment.

## Tip 4. Make OCD the Problem, Not Your Child

Reinforce this message with your child. One way to do this is to call OCD by the nasty nickname your child chooses to give it in Session 2. (Adolescents commonly just call OCD by its medical name.) In this way, OCD becomes the "bad guy" while you and your child are the "good guys" who are working to make OCD "get out of Dodge." When you're tempted to view your child's OCD symptoms as bad behavior, remember that OCD is an illness and that your youngster is sick. Criticism and other forms of punishment make it harder to resist OCD, so work to practice generosity, kindness, and most of all, patience while you and your child's therapist implement the treatment strategies that will, in the long run, reduce OCD symptoms.

## Tip 5. The Therapist Is Your Child's Coach

Once OCD is clearly identified and named as the problem, the difficult process of "bossing back" OCD begins. The nugget at the heart of "bossing back" OCD is exposure and response prevention (E/RP), with the therapist serving as "coach" to facilitate that E/RP. *Exposure* occurs when the child exposes himself or herself to the feared object, action, or thought. *Response prevention* is the process of blocking the rituals and/or minimizing the avoidance behaviors that result from exposure. With exposure and response prevention, anxiety over the obsession and associated rituals decreases or even disappears. Take, for example, the child with a contamination fear about touching doorknobs. In this case, since doorknobs trigger the obsession, the exposure task would be for the child to hold the "contaminated" doorknob. Next, response prevention takes place when the child refuses to perform the usual anxiety-driven compulsion, such as washing hands or using a tissue to grasp the knob. During therapy sessions, the therapist and the child together decide on an E/RP task to be practiced daily between sessions. Not surprisingly, E/RP must be carefully structured so that your child will want to stick with treatment. This treatment program includes very specific ways for ensuring that E/RP leads to decreases in OCD symptoms. Implementing E/RP is the job of your child's therapist, who coaches your child in the strategies for winning the contest with OCD. Just as you wouldn't tell your child's basketball coach how to coach basketball, the structure of CBT for OCD must of necessity remain under the control of your child's therapist. If you have questions about how things are going, please ask your therapist before a little problem becomes a big one, but remember that your job is to support your child, not to coach.

## Tip 6. Stop Giving Advice

For the most part, children already know that OCD makes no sense. Thus, reminding the child that his or her behavior is crazy, goofy, or nonsensical usually just makes the child feel bad. Similarly, advice to "just stop it" has the same effect; no one hates OCD more than the child who has it. He or she would have stopped already, if possible. Often, OCD causes problems in some places but not others, or at one time and not another, which not unreasonably causes parents to think that OCD is willful misbehavior. For example, a child may be able to use one bathroom in the house or not another, or may be fine with bathrooms at home but not at school. Remember that it is the nature of OCD *not* to make sense, and don't misinterpret the unevenness of OCD symptoms as calling for well-intentioned advice or injunctions to cease and desist.

## Tip 7. Be a Cheerleader for Your Child

As a cheerleader, you can help motivate your child as he or she begins to boss back OCD. By exhibiting a supportive and confidently neutral attitude, you can help reduce your child's anxiety during exposure tasks. Criticism or punishment invariably makes OCD worse by decreasing your child's motivation to resist. Remember that you wouldn't criticize your youngster for having asthma; OCD is not much different. Remember also that the tasks chosen for E/RP may seem small and insignificant, but it is important for E/RP to take place at your child's pace.

## Tip 8. Learn All You Can about OCD

If you had asthma, diabetes, or heart disease, you'd want to know as much about your illness and its treatment as possible. The same is true for OCD. Fortunately, there are many resources that can help you with this task, including lay and professional books, the OC Foundation, the OC Information Center, and even OCD sites on the Internet. We especially encourage you to join the OC Foundation, which supports patients and families struggling with OCD, and also works to expand knowledge about OCD by disseminating information and supporting research into the cause and cure of OCD.

## THE "TOOL KIT"

Your child is now learning about what we call a "tool kit" to use during trial exposure and response prevention (E/RP) tasks. This tool kit consists of specific techniques your child can use to cope with the anxiety that comes from trial E/RP homework. You may encourage and remind your child to try using his or her tool kit when doing the weekly homework. While these techniques may come into play spontaneously with other OCD thoughts or urges, it is not helpful to insist that your child use these techniques in an area of OCD that your child is not yet ready to resist. The tool kit can be used, however, any time your child is experiencing anxiety. The tool kit consists of a "map" of your child's OCD, a "fear thermometer" for grading feelings during E/RP, and cognitive strategies for "talking back" to OCD. Depending on the nature of your child's symptoms, some children may also be taught anxiety reducing techniques, such as diaphragmatic breathing and muscle relaxation.

## Tip 9. When You Are Trying to Understand How Your Child Feels, Use the Fear Thermometer

The fear thermometer, which rates anxiety from 1 (none) to 10 (intolerable panic), provides the child with a tool for measuring anxiety or other uncomfortable feelings. The fear thermometer uses a numerical scale to help the child rank specific OCD symptoms with respect to their potency or difficulty when presented as targets for E/RP. The fear thermometer is also used during exposure tasks to measure the child's anxiety until it diminishes, thus documenting the success of the treatment strategy. Additionally, the fear thermometer helps the child be more realistic about his or her probable responses to OCD triggers: All fear isn't absolute terror. Since OCD fears decrease with treatment, fear thermometer ratings change over time. With the therapist's help, fear thermometer ratings can become a way for you and your child to communicate about the degree to which OCD causes fear and upset. The fear thermometer is also an important key to generating an detailed map of OCD.

## Tip 10. Contribute to Your Child's Map of OCD

Having first itemized all the OCD symptoms—triggers, obsessions, and corresponding compulsions—that bother your child, the therapist will help your child learn to rank these OCD symptoms from the easiest to the hardest to "boss back" using the fear thermometer. You'll want to contribute to this process by making sure that the list includes OCD symptoms that tangle you up as well as your child. Having ranked OCD symptoms, it is straightforward to understand where the child's life territory is free from OCD, where OCD and the child each "win" some of the time, and where the child yields control to OCD. We call the region where the child is sometimes able to successfully "boss back" OCD the *transition or work zone* (see Handout 2). As treatment proceeds, the transition/work zone provides a dependable guide for the child to use when selecting targets for graded E/RP. In this way, the map metaphor leads to the concept of a *symptom list* or *stimulus hierarchy*, that is, a list of OC symptoms ranked according to the difficulty they present for exposure and response prevention. The "map" and stimulus hierarchy also help to project into the future how the child will move up the hierarchy from easy to more difficult elements. If you understand the stimulus hierarchy and know what E/RP targets have been selected or not selected for homework, you'll be able to tell when to encourage and when to practice patience relative to your child's' OCD symptoms.

## Tip 11. Encourage Constructive Self-Talk

Encourage your child to speak positively but realistically about his efforts to resist OCD. Most children with OCD are very critical of themselves for engaging in rituals, especially when doing so causes failure in school or problems at home. Negative self-talk contributes to the overall anxiety experienced before, during, and after exposure tasks. Identifying and correcting negative self-talk is crucial to increasing motivation for E/RP. The general approach relies on replacing maladaptive cognitions—either overly optimistic or pessimistic—with realistic self-statements that emphasize the child's ability to cope with OCD using the tools taught in treatment. Take, for example, a youngster with contamination fears and washing rituals who chooses to decrease her usual 2-hour shower by 15 minutes as a homework task. If her internal self-statements prior to the exposure task are: "I won't be able to do this. What if I take an even longer shower?" then the likelihood of her actually attempting the exposure task decreases significantly. To decrease the child's general anxiety and increase motivation to practice the exposure task, she might consciously think: "This task will be difficult, but I can handle this much anxiety this one time. I'll use my tool kit."

## Tip 12. Talk Back to OCD

Another form of constructive self-talk is made possible by the effort to externalize OCD (make OCD the problem separate from the child). This involves the child's conversation with OCD itself, which we call "talking back to OCD." You and you child can refuse to give in to OCD, talking back to it in a positive forceful fashion, thereby keeping OCD external to the child and increasing the child's motivation to comply with E/RP. Bossing back OCD in conversation can be difficult, especially when the child directly challenges obsessions with statements that themselves can cause OCD symptoms, such as, "I won't get sick if I touch this faucet." Under these circumstances, it is sometimes helpful to suggest that the child use more general "talking back " strategies, such as, "Go jump in the lake OCD, I'm the boss" or "Can't catch me this time, OCD." When bossing back OCD, it is important to do so only for targets that have been selected as homework during the current week or earlier weeks. Otherwise, you'll be encouraging your child to do the impossible—namely, tackle targets that are still too high on the stimulus hierarchy.

Tip 13: Encourage Accurate Risk Appraisal

OCD symptoms that are driven by fear, guilt, or disgust often involve overestimation of the likelihood that a terrible event will occur, the cost of the event in question, or an exaggerated sense of personal responsibility for the dread outcome. For example, a child might have a hateful thought, which provokes the obsession that he and his family will go to hell, which in turn causes the child to engage in praying rituals to relieve the obsession and accompanying anxiety. In this example, the child behaves as though the trigger (the hateful thought) has a 100% chance of causing an adverse consequence (hell), which will be catastrophic, and that he alone is responsible for the dread outcome. This is the origin of the many conversations you've probably had about the senseless or unreasonable nature of OCD. While it is not helpful to argue about whether rituals are necessary or not, it is possible, under the direction of your child's therapist, to help your child realistically estimate the danger of the dreaded outcomes. The first part of this process involves analyzing how OCD encourages catastrophic thinking. The second looks at how the child exaggerates his or her sense of responsibility for the occurrence of the catastrophe event. In both, the faulty assumptions underlying obsessions are directly confronted, first by the therapist in conversation with the child, and later by the child with OCD during E/RP tasks. Using his or her cognitive analytic abilities to generate a "proof" that OCD is speaking nonsense, your child should be more willing to try an exposure task to verify the prediction that nothing bad will indeed happen if he or she does the opposite of what OCD requires. Having learned this process along with your child, you can also encourage your child to be realistic about danger without hammering away on the unreasonableness of OCD.

Tip 14: Cultivate a Sense of Detachment from OCD

Confronting OCD through "talking back" or cognitive restructuring involves taking OCD on its own terms. An alternative strategy, popularized by Jeff Schwartz in his book Brain Lock (HarperCollins, 1996), relies on cultivating detachment from OCD. Cultivating detachment meshes very nicely with narrative approaches to externalizing the problem, such as giving OCD a nasty nickname, and is especially helpful for those patients who tend to lose perspective when they become anxious. The basic idea is simple: OCD is just a brain hiccup that comes and goes in its own time, so we ask patients to see OCD as though it is "just a cloud in the sky," "a fish swimming by in an aquarium," or "a bunch of crazy monkeys up in a tree."

Working with OCD in this fashion involves teaching the child four simple self-statements to use when OCD makes an appearance. First, the child says something like "It's just OCD again," recognizing that the obsessions are OCD and are not meaningful self-statements. Sometimes, generating a friendly "Hi [whatever nickname the child has chosen for OCD]" helps reduce the child's tendency to react emotionally to the OCD symptoms. Second, the child states, "My brain is hiccuping again," explicitly recognizing that what we call OCD arises because of misfiring central nervous system circuits. Third, the child comments, "These hiccups are not in themselves important," implying that no response other than patient endurance is necessary because the content of OCD is meaningless. Finally, given meaningless symptoms that will pass away on their own if nothing is done, the child says, "I guess I'll go do something pleasant while OCD goes away." Cultivating detachment will help you avoid getting upset with the inconvenience caused by OCD. Even better, while waiting for OCD to disappear, you and your child can do something more enjoyable together, such as reading a story, taking a walk, or playing a game.

## Tip 15. Encourage Your Child to Use the Short Form of Cognitive Training during E/RP

Most children end up merging parts of all three techniques: "bossing back," cognitive restructuring, and cultivating detachment. Having settled on what is most acceptable and useful for a particular youngster, we usually provide a specific step-by-step strategy for thinking about OCD when doing an exposure task. For some children, it is helpful to list the steps on a 3" × 5" card that can be used during E/RP. For example, your child might notice that she has been worrying about whether or not she can touch a certain doorknob. Step one would be to tell herself that this worry is simply OCD, distinguishing between the obsession (her mother will get sick) and the compulsion (avoiding her mother and washing). Step two would be to remind herself that she doesn't have to pay any attention to OCD; it's just her brain playing tricks on her. Step three involves reminding herself that the discomfort she experiences when touching the doorknob will go away in a little while so that she doesn't need to do the ritual. Step four is to choose to focus her thoughts and/or actions on something besides OCD, such as the soccer game she will play that afternoon, while she waits for the OCD symptoms to abate. Under the direction of your child's therapist, you can help encourage your youngster to use the cognitive tool kit to more skillfully manage his or her response to OCD.

## Tip 16. Rewards

Unlike the treatment of attention-deficit/hyperactivity disorder (ADHD), the treatment of OCD doesn't rely on teaching parents how to issue effective commands or to punish bad or reward good behavior. On the other hand, positive reinforcement can be quite helpful in increasing the motivation to resist OCD, especially for the youngster who has been exposed to a steady stream of negative comments or punishment because of OCD symptoms. Your therapist will help you negotiate a set of rewards for successfully "bossing back OCD" in the form of small prizes or treats. Rewards for specific tasks also help keep the focus on OCD as the problem, while at the same time increasing your child's self-esteem and motivation. You should not think of these rewards as "bribery." Resisting OCD is hard work and it is reasonable to reward it just like any other chore.

## HELPING YOUR CHILD "BOSS BACK" OCD

Parents are almost always consciously supportive of the child with OCD. However, since OCD didn't come with an owner's guide, parents also find themselves unwittingly supporting OCD. In order for the child to make progress against OCD, you must learn how to disengage yourself from OCD, and become wholly supportive of your child. You can play one of several roles with respect to OCD: (1) OCD's *helper* (a nontherapeutic role, and one to be written out of the child's story); (2) *cheerleader* for the child; and (3) *cotherapist* (usually with the child's permission). Obviously, we want to discourage the first, encourage the second, and carefully structure the third. Making these changes in a way that keeps everyone—child, parent, and therapist—successfully aligned against OCD isn't easy. For example, a parent who ceases to provide reassurance about a contamination fear explicitly generates a response prevention task for the child. Thus, all changes in parental behavior relative to OCD must first be screened for their location on the stimulus hierarchy and, if possible, should always be implemented with the child's assent. Your therapist will structure your involvement to be sure that things go as smoothly as possible.

### Tip 17. Don't Be a Helper

Parents, family members, and friends are often brought into the child's rituals and so become entangled in OCD's territory. It is important to identify the ways OCD bosses you around, since withdrawing your support from OCD is one key to successful treatment. This is why your child's therapist needs your input about the nature of your child's OCD symptoms, especially those rituals that involve people besides the child. We involve parents in the treatment process by helping the parents and child decide *together* how the parents will no longer participate in OCD. This requires that the child choose targets for parental E/RP, and that the therapist provide specific "coaching" for family members who will be participating in these E/RP tasks. For example, parents often wish "no matter what" to stop participating in certain rituals, despite the fact that doing so would cause great distress in the child that the parents might be unable to manage. The trick is to move up the symptom hierarchy at the child's pace, letting the child choose how to withdraw parents from the role of OCD's helper. For example, the child may ask the parent to help keep the water turned off while he or she is performing a contamination-related exposure task. Doing so explicitly changes the parent's role from one of OCD's helper to one of cheerleader and, eventually, to cotherapist/coach.

### Tip 18. Cheerleading Is a Great Way to Help Your Child Boss Back OCD

Until your child is ready to enlist you as a cotherapist, your role as cheerleader is to offer support and encouragement. This will contribute to your child's confidence as he or she tackles the E/RP homework. Just as cheerleaders cheer *only* the play at hand, so you should cheer your child on to complete *only* the homework task at hand and not pressure him or her to attempt things that are as yet too difficult.

### Tip 19. As Cotherapist or Coach You Assist Your Child in the Homework Task

With your child's prior permission, and with specific coaching from the therapist, parents can sometimes be a great help by acting as cotherapists. This is especially important for difficult E/RP tasks that are located at some distance from the office setting so that your child's therapist can't be there to help out. For example, your child may ask you to keep the water turned off while he or she is performing a contamination task in the bathroom at home. While your child is waiting for his anxiety to decrease, you can offer encouragement from the sidelines by saying, "There goes OCD trying to boss you around again. Remember the anxious feeling will go away. You can do it! Just use your tool kit." In addition, you can ask your child about their temperature on the fear temperature at 1- to 2-minute intervals so that your child can "see" his or her fear decreasing.

### Tip 20. More Rewards, Ceremonies, and Notifications

Ceremonies (symbolic tokens of achievement) and notifications (letting other people know about your child's successes in getting better) are tangible reminders that OCD is being bossed out of your child's story. Ceremonies, like other rewards, are morale boosters; notifications help others, who may previously have considered the youngster to be badly behaved, recognize that he or she is actually working very hard to recover from a difficult mental illness. Together with your child and the therapist, you can help identify those goals that, when reached, will be celebrated with rewards, ceremonies, and notifications.

### Tip 21. Keeping Up with the Map

During the next parent session, we will focus specifically on response prevention tasks that you as parents may choose with the agreement of your child. Until then, observe and identify any territory where OCD makes you its helper. Make a written list of these situations in order of difficulty and bring the list to each session so that the therapist can incorporate these targets in the symptom hierarchy. Your child will continue to tackle E/RP over the next 6 weeks, and will greatly benefit from your role as cheerleader, or, if you are asked, as cotherapist and coach.

### KEEPING UP WITH EXPOSURE AND RESPONSE PREVENTION: CHOOSING THE COTHERAPIST ROLE

In today's parent session, we spoke about specific ways you as parents can act as your child's cotherapist by saying no to the ways OCD actually bosses you around. When you stop being "bossed" by OCD, your child will feel the effects as an exposure task. During today's session, you and your child decided on one ritual you will no longer participate in this week. The following are suggestions and reminders of ways you can respond to the anxiety your child will experience as you no longer do what OCD requires.

### Tip 22. Reiterate the Agreement

When your child insists on your participation in the specified ritual, remind him or her that you are not going to let OCD be the boss in this situation.

### Tip 23. Encourage Your Child to Stick with It

Encourage your child to use his or her tool kit to stick with it, reminding him that bailing out on OCD (escape/avoidance) is the best way to be sure that OCD hangs around.

## Tip 24. Use the Fear Thermometer

Check on your child's level of anxiety and encourage him or her to use the fear thermometer.

## Tip 25. Be a Cheerleader

Congratulate your child when your refusal to participate in the ritual no longer produces anxiety. Set up rewards, ceremonies, and notifications that are appropriate to the challenges your child faces. A new ritual can be targeted each week as everyone agrees on the next challenge. The coaching process is the same each time, although different strategies may be chosen according to your child's needs. Remember that you must work on the E/RP targets decided upon with your child and the therapist. Premature E/RP inhibits progress by taking the wind out of your child's sails and reducing his or her motivation to cooperate with treatment.

## Tip 26. Don't Abruptly Stop Participating in Rituals

When extensive family involvement in rituals requires that family members play a central role in treatment, take direction from the therapist about when to cooperate and when to stop cooperating with rituals. Abruptly stopping your participation in OCD rituals without your child's consent is almost never helpful, since neither you nor your child will have a workable strategy for managing the resulting distress; it won't reduce those symptoms that are out of sight, and, most importantly, you won't be helping your child internalize a lifelong strategy for coping with current and potential OCD symptoms.

## Tip 27. What Should I Do When I or My Child Feels Like Quitting?

It is normal to have occasional doubts and discomfort with treatment. Be sure to discuss all your concerns and any discomforts with your doctor, therapist, and other family members. If you feel a treatment is not working or is causing unpleasant side effects, tell your doctor—don't stop CBT or adjust your medication on your own. It is harder to get OCD under control than to keep it there, so don't risk relapse by discontinuing treatment without first consulting your doctor and cognitive-behavioral therapist. Also, if things aren't going well, don't be shy about asking for a second opinion from another clinician who is an expert in the treatment of OCD. Consultations with an expert in medication management or in behavioral psychotherapy can be a great help.

## RELAPSE PREVENTION

Congratulations! OCD now has only a small role in your child's life. To keep it that way, your child has learned some relapse prevention strategies to deal with the occasional OCD hiccup. This week, your child will choose an exposure task in which he or she feels OCD is most likely to try and make a "comeback." The following tips can be used when OCD tries to reclaim territory.

### Tip 28. Use E/RP on Purpose

When an OCD urge or hiccup comes, encourage your child to *boss it back with an intentional exposure task*, using the tool kit to manage anxiety. The idea here is to do the opposite of what OCD tells you to do *right away*. For example, if your child has a thought about burning the house down if he or she doesn't check the toaster, encourage him to walk over to the toaster, look at the plug once for a few seconds, and then walk away.

### Tip 29. Avoid Avoidance

Often an OCD hiccup comes in the form of avoidance, which may seem harmless or difficult to detect at first. It is important to confront these situations immediately, so that OCD cannot secretly take back territory that your child now claims.

### Tip 30. Practice E/RP

When a hiccup occurs, encourage your child to practice the corresponding exposure task each day for a week, or until it no longer produces any anxiety.

### Tip 31. Continue to Be a Cheerleader for Your Child

OCD can a difficult disease that waxes and wanes, despite our best intentions. As a result, OCD requires ongoing monitoring. Children, particularly adolescents, can become discouraged by the long-term nature of OCD, even when they have very few, if any, symptoms. Remind your child that bossing back OCD in any way is a sign of his or her own personal strength and courage. Remember also, there are far worse illnesses than OCD, and that he or she can grow up to have a full and satisfying life despite OCD.

## WHEN TREATMENT ENDS

### Tip 32. How Often Should I Talk with My Child's Doctor?

At the beginning of treatment, most families and patients talk with their doctor at least once a week to monitor symptoms, medication doses, and side effects. As your child recovers, contact becomes less frequent; once well, he or she might see the doctor for a quick review every few months for the first year, and once a year after that.

### Tip 33. Regardless of Scheduled Appointments or Blood Tests, Call the Doctor If Your Child Has the Following:

- Recurrent severe OCD symptoms that come out of nowhere.
- Worsening OCD symptoms that don't respond to strategies learned in CBT.
- Changes in medication side effects.
- New symptoms of another disorder, such as panic disorder or depression.
- A life event, such as a school crisis, that might worsen OCD.

### Tip 34. What about the Rest of My Child's Life?

While your child is working hard to get better, let him approach life at his or her own pace. Avoid the extremes of expecting too much or too little. Don't push too hard. Remember that nobody hates OCD more than the patient, so be supportive rather than critical of his or her efforts to resist OCD. A thoughtful patient attitude is especially important with respect to school work. Since OCD often results in a temporary decrease in school performance, be patient even if much of the school year turns out to be a less than ideal experience academically. Remember, your child is ill. You (and the school) would take a kindly approach if you were dealing with asthma or diabetes— why not with OCD? Depending on necessity, your therapist will help you work with the school, so that they become part of the treatment team.

### Tip 35. What If My Child Won't Talk to Me?

If your child views your concern as interference and doesn't want to talk to you about whether OCD is still hanging around, remember that this is not a rejection of you—it is either the illness talking, in which case it will become obvious when OCD reaches a clinical level of severity, or it is just one of those developmental stages that children go through, in which case it is nothing to worry about. If you are unsure, a call to the therapist may help you decide if an office visit is needed. In general, however, it is best to treat your child normally once she has recovered, while remaining alert for telltale symptoms. Learn, however, to tell the difference between a bad day and OCD. Don't attribute everything that goes poorly to OCD.

## Tip 36. Taking Care of Yourself

If you are helping to care for someone with severe OCD at home, try, if possible, to take turns "checking in" on your child's needs so that OCD doesn't overburden one family member. Another way of sharing the burden, as well as getting more useful tips about how to manage OCD, is to join a support group. The OC Foundation will tell you if a support group is available in your area. Support groups are also available on the Internet.

# Expert Consensus Treatment Guidelines for Obsessive–Compulsive Disorder: A Guide for Patients and Families

If you or someone you care about has been diagnosed with obsessive–compulsive disorder (OCD), you may feel you are the only person facing the difficulties of this illness. But you are not alone. In the United States, 1 in 50 adults currently has OCD, and twice that many have had it at some point in their lives. Fortunately, very effective treatments for OCD are now available to help you regain a more satisfying life. Here are answers to the most commonly asked questions about OCD.

## WHAT IS OBSESSIVE–COMPULSIVE DISORDER?

Worries, doubts, superstitious beliefs—all are common in everyday life. However, when they become so excessive—such as hours of hand washing—or make no sense at all—such as driving around and around the block to check that an accident didn't occur—then a diagnosis of OCD is made. In OCD, it is as though the brain gets stuck on a particular thought or urge and just can't let go. People with OCD often say the symptoms feel like a case of mental hiccups that won't go away. OCD is a medical brain disorder that causes problems in information processing. It is not your fault or the result of a "weak" or unstable personality. Before the arrival of modern medications and cognitive-behavioral therapy, OCD was generally thought to be untreatable. Most people with OCD continued to suffer, despite years of ineffective psychotherapy. Today, luckily, treatment can help most people with OCD. Although OCD is usually completely curable only in some individuals, most people achieve meaningful symptom relief with comprehensive treatment.

This guide was prepared with the help of the Obsessive–Compulsive Foundation and includes recommendations contained in the *Expert Consensus Treatment Guidelines for Obsessive–Compulsive Disorder*. The Expert Consensus Treatment Guidelines Project for Obsessive–Compulsive Disorder was supported by an unrestricted educational grant from Solvay Pharmaceuticals. From March, Frances, et al. (1997). Copyright 1997 by Expert Knowledge Systems, LLC. Reprinted by permission in *OCD in Children and Adolescents: A Cognitive-Behavioral Treatment Manual* by John S. March and Karen Mulle. Permission to photocopy this handout is granted to purchasers of *OCD in Children and Adolescents* for personal use only (see copyright page for details).

The successful treatment of OCD, just like that of other medical disorders, requires certain changes in behavior and sometimes medication.

## What Are the Symptoms of Obsessive–Compulsive Disorder?

OCD usually involves having both obsessions and compulsions, though a person with OCD may sometimes have only one or the other. Table 1 lists some common obsessions and compulsions. OCD symptoms can occur in people of all ages. Not all obsessive–compulsive behaviors represent an illness. Some rituals (e.g., bedtime songs, religious practices) are a welcome part of daily life. Normal worries, such as contamination fears, may increase during times of stress, such as when someone in the family is sick or dying. Only when symptoms persist, make no sense, cause much distress, or interfere with functioning do they need clinical attention.

1. *Obsessions*. Obsessions are thoughts, images, or impulses that occur over and over again and feel out of your control. The person does not want to have these ideas, finds them disturbing and intrusive, and usually recognizes that they don't really make sense. People with OCD may worry excessively about dirt and germs and be obsessed with the idea that they are contaminated or may contaminate others. Or they may have obsessive fears of having inadvertently harmed someone else (perhaps while pulling the car out of the driveway), even though they usually know this is not realistic. Obsessions are

**TABLE 1.** Typical OCD Symptoms

| Common obsessions | Common compulsions |
|---|---|
| • Contamination fears of germs, dirt, etc. | • Washing |
| • Imagining having harmed self or others | • Repeating |
| • Imagining losing control of aggressive urges | • Checking |
| • Intrusive sexual thoughts or urges | • Touching |
| • Excessive religious or moral doubt | • Counting |
| • Forbidden thoughts | • Ordering/arranging |
| • A need to have things "just so" | • Hoarding or saving |
| • A need to tell, ask, confess | • Praying |

accompanied by uncomfortable feelings, such as fear, disgust, doubt, or a sensation that things have to be done in a way that is "just so."

2. *Compulsions*. People with OCD typically try to make their obsessions go away by performing compulsions. Compulsions are acts the person performs over and over again, often according to certain "rules." People with an obsession about contamination may wash constantly to the point that their hands become raw and inflamed. A person may repeatedly check that she has turned off the stove or iron because of an obsessive fear of burning the house down. She may have to count certain objects over and over because of an obsession about losing them. Unlike compulsive drinking or gambling, OCD compulsions do not give the person pleasure. Rather, the rituals are performed to obtain relief from the discomfort caused by the obsessions.

3. *Other features of obsessive–compulsive disorder.*

- OCD symptoms cause distress, take up a lot of time (more than an hour a day), or significantly interfere with the person's work, social life, or relationships.
- Most individuals with OCD recognize at some point that their obsessions are coming from within their own minds and are not just excessive worries about real problems, and that the compulsions they perform are excessive or unreasonable. When someone with OCD does not recognize that their beliefs and actions are unreasonable, this is called OCD with poor insight.
- OCD symptoms tend to wax and wane over time. Some may be little more than background noise; others may produce extremely severe distress.

## When Does Obsessive–Compulsive Disorder Begin?

OCD can start at any time from preschool age to adulthood (usually by age 40). One-third to one-half of adults with OCD report that it started during childhood. Unfortunately, OCD often goes unrecognized. On average, people with OCD see three to four doctors and spend over 9 years seeking treatment before they receive a correct diagnosis. Studies have also found that it takes an average of 17 years from the time OCD begins for people to obtain appropriate treatment. OCD tends to be underdiagnosed and undertreated for a number of reasons. People with OCD may be secretive about their symptoms or lack insight about their illness. Many healthcare providers are not familiar with the symptoms or are not trained in providing the appropriate treatments.

Some people may not have access to treatment resources. This is unfortunate since earlier diagnosis and proper treatment, including finding the right medications, can help people avoid the suffering associated with OCD and lessen the risk of developing other problems, such as depression or marital and work problems.

## Is Obsessive–Compulsive Disorder Inherited?

No specific genes for OCD have yet been identified, but research suggests that genes do play a role in the development of the disorder in some cases. Childhood-onset OCD tends to run in families (sometimes in association with tic disorders).When a parent has OCD, there is a slightly increased risk that a child will develop OCD, although the risk is still low. When OCD runs in families, it is the general nature of OCD that seems to be inherited, not specific symptoms. Thus a child may have checking rituals, while his mother washes compulsively.

## What Causes Obsessive–Compulsive Disorder?

There is no single, proven cause of OCD. Research suggests that OCD involves problems in communication between the front part of the brain (the orbital cortex) and deeper structures (the basal ganglia). These brain structures use the chemical messenger serotonin. It is believed that insufficient levels of serotonin are prominently involved in OCD. Drugs that increase the brain concentration of serotonin often help improve OCD symptoms. Pictures of the brain at work also show that the brain circuits involved in OCD return toward normal in those who improve after taking a serotonin medication or receiving cognitive-behavioral psychotherapy. Although it seems clear that reduced levels of serotonin play a role in OCD, there is no laboratory test for OCD. Rather, the diagnosis is made based on an assessment of the person's symptoms. When OCD starts suddenly in childhood in association with strep throat, an autoimmune mechanism may be involved, and treatment with an antibiotic may prove helpful.

## What Other Problems Are Sometimes Confused with OCD?

- Some disorders that closely resemble OCD and may respond to some of the same treatments are trichotillomania (compulsive hair pulling), body dysmorphic disorder (imagined ugliness), and habit disorders, such as nail biting or skin picking. While they share superficial similarities, impulse control problems, such as substance abuse, pathological gambling, or compulsive sexual activity are probably not related to OCD in any substantial way.

• The most common conditions that resemble OCD are the tic disorders (Tourette's Disorder and other motor and vocal tic disorders). Tics are involuntary motor behaviors (such as facial grimacing) or vocal behaviors (such as snorting) that often occur in response to a feeling of discomfort. More complex tics, like touching or tapping tics, may closely resemble compulsions. Tics and OCD occur together much more often when the OCD or tics begin during childhood.

• Depression and OCD often occur together in adults and, less commonly, in children and adolescents. However, unless depression is also present, people with OCD are not generally sad or lacking in pleasure, and people who are depressed but do not have OCD rarely have the kinds of intrusive thoughts that are characteristic of OCD.

• Although stress can make OCD worse, most people with OCD report that the symptoms can come and go on their own. OCD is easy to distinguish from a condition called posttraumatic stress disorder, because OCD is not caused by a terrible event.

• Schizophrenia, delusional disorders, and other psychotic conditions are usually easy to distinguish from OCD. Unlike psychotic individuals, people with OCD continue to have a clear idea of what is real and what is not.

• In children and adolescents, OCD may worsen or cause disruptive behaviors, exaggerate a preexisting learning disorder, cause problems with attention and concentration, or interfere with learning at school. In many children with OCD, these disruptive behaviors are related to the OCD and will go away when the OCD is successfully treated.

• Individuals with OCD may have substance-abuse problems, sometimes as a result of attempts to self-medicate. Specific treatment for the substance abuse is usually also needed.

• Children and adults with pervasive developmental disorders (autism, Asperger's disorder) are extremely rigid and compulsive, with stereotyped behaviors that somewhat resemble very severe OCD. However, those with pervasive developmental disorders have extremely severe problems relating to and communicating with other people, which do not occur in OCD.

Only a small number of those with OCD have the collection of personality traits called obsessive compulsive personality disorder (OCPD). Despite its similar name, OCPD does not involve obsessions and compulsions, but rather is a personality pattern that involves a preoccupation with rules, schedules, and lists and characteristic traits such as perfectionism, an excessive devotion to work, rigidity, and inflexibility. However, when people have both OCPD and OCD, the successful treatment of the OCD often causes a favorable change in the person's personality.

## HOW IS OBSESSIVE–COMPULSIVE DISORDER TREATED?

The first step in treating OCD is educating the patient and family about OCD and its treatment as a medical illness. During the last 20 years, two effective treatments for OCD have been developed: *cognitive-behavioral psychotherapy* (CBT) and medication with a *serotonin reuptake inhibitor* (SRI).

### Stages of Treatment

- Acute treatment phase: Treatment is aimed at ending the current episode of OCD.
- Maintenance treatment: Treatment is aimed at preventing future episodes of OCD.

### Components of Treatment

- Education: crucial in helping patients and families learn how best to manage OCD and prevent its complications.
- Psychotherapy: Cognitive-behavioral psychotherapy (CBT) is the key element of treatment for most patients with OCD.
- Medication: Medication with a serotonin reuptake inhibitor is helpful for many patients.

## EDUCATION

### Is There Anything I Can Do to Help My Disorder?

Absolutely yes. You need to become an expert on your illness. Since OCD can come and go many times during your life, you and your family or others close to you need to learn all about OCD and its treatment. This will help you get the best treatment and keep the illness under control. Read books, attend lectures, talk to your doctor or therapist, and consider joining the Obsessive–Compulsive Foundation. A list of recommended readings and information resources is given at the end of this handout. Being an informed patient is the surest path to success.

## How Often Should I Talk with My Clinician?

When beginning treatment, most people talk to their clinician at least once a week to develop a CBT treatment plan and to monitor symptoms, medication doses, and side effects. As you get better, you see your clinician less often. Once you are well, you might see your clinician only once a year.

Regardless of scheduled appointments or blood tests, call your clinician if you have:

- Recurrent severe OCD symptoms that come out-of-nowhere
- Worsening OCD symptoms that don't respond to strategies you learned in CBT
- Changes in medication side effects
- New symptoms of another disorder (e.g., panic or depression)
- A crisis (e.g., a job change) that might worsen your OCD.

## What Should I Do If I Feel Like Quitting Treatment?

It is normal to have occasional doubts and discomfort with your treatment. Discuss your concerns and any discomforts with your doctor, therapist, and family. If you feel a medication is not working or is causing unpleasant side effects, tell your doctor. Don't stop or adjust your medication on your own. You and your doctor can work together to find the best and most comfortable medicine for you. Also, don't be shy about asking for a second opinion from another clinician, especially about the wisdom of cognitive-behavior therapy. Consultations with an expert on medication or behavioral psychotherapy can be a great help. *Remember, it is harder to get OCD under control than to keep it there, so don't risk a relapse by stopping your treatment without first talking to your clinician.*

## What Can Families and Friends Do to Help?

- Many family members feel frustrated and confused by the symptoms of OCD. They don't know how to help their loved one. If you are a family member or friend of someone with OCD, your first and most important task is to learn as much as you can about the disorder, its causes, and its treatment. At the same time, you must be sure the person with OCD has access to information about the disorder. We highly recommend the booklet, "Learning to Live with Obsessive Compulsive Disorder" by Van Noppen et al. (Information on obtaining this and other educational resources is given at the end of this handout.) This booklet gives good advice and practical tips to help family members help their loved ones and learn to cope with OCD. Helping the person to understand that there are treatments that can help is a big step toward getting the person into treatment. When a person with OCD denies that there is a problem or refuses to go for treatment, this can be very difficult for family members. Continue to offer educational materials to the person. In some cases. it may help to hold a family meeting to discuss the problem, in a similar manner to what is often done when someone with alcohol problems is in denial.

• Family problems don't cause OCD, but the way families react to the symptoms can affect the disorder, just as the symptoms can cause a great deal of disruption and many problems for the family. OCD rituals can tangle up family members unmercifully, and it is sometimes necessary for the family to go through therapy with the patient. The therapist can help family members learn how to become gradually disentangled from the rituals in small steps and with the patient's agreement. Abruptly stopping your participation in OCD rituals without the patient's consent is rarely helpful since you and the patient will not know how to manage the distress that results. Your refusal to participate will not help with those symptoms that are hidden and, most important, will not help the patient learn a lifelong strategy for coping with OCD symptoms.

• Negative comments or criticism from family members often make OCD worse, while a calm, supportive family can help improve the outcome of treatment. If the person views your help as interference, remember it is the illness talking. Try to be as kind and patient as possible since this is the best way to help get rid of the OCD symptoms. Telling someone with OCD to simply stop their compulsive behaviors usually doesn't help and can make the person feel worse, since he or she is not able to comply. Instead, praise any successful attempts to resist OCD, while focusing your attention on positive elements in the person's life. You must avoid expecting too much or too little. Don't push too hard. Remember that nobody hates OCD more than the person who has the disorder. Treat people normally once they have recovered, but be alert for telltale signs of relapse. If the illness is starting to come back, you may notice it before the person does. Point out the early symptoms in a caring manner and suggest a discussion with the doctor. Learn to tell the difference between a bad day and OCD, however. It is important not to attribute everything that goes poorly to OCD.

• Family members can help the clinician treat the patient. When your family member is in treatment, talk with the clinician if possible. You could offer to visit the clinician with the person to share your observations about how the treatment is going. Encourage the patient to stick with medications and/or CBT. However, if the patient has been on a certain treatment for a fairly long time with little improvement in symptoms or has troubling side effects, encourage the person to ask the doctor about other treatments or about getting a second opinion.

• When children or adolescents have OCD, it is important for parents to work with schools and teachers to be sure that they understand the disorder. Just as with any child with an illness, parents still need to set consistent limits and let the child or adolescent know what is expected of him or her.

• Take advantage of the help available from support groups (for addresses and phone numbers, see the end of this handout). Sharing your worries and experiences with others who have gone through the same things can be a big help. Support groups are a good way to feel less alone and to learn new strategies for coping and helping the person with OCD.

• Be sure to make time for yourself and your own life. If you are helping to care for someone with severe OCD at home, try to take turns "checking in" on the person so that no one family member or friend bears too much of the burden. It is important to continue to lead your own life and not let yourself become a prisoner of your loved one's rituals. You will then be better able to provide support for your loved one.

## PSYCHOTHERAPY

Cognitive-behavioral therapy (CBT) is the psychotherapeutic treatment of choice for children, adolescents, and adults with OCD. In CBT, there is a logically consistent and compelling relationship between the disorder, the treatment, and the desired outcome. CBT helps the patient internalize a strategy for resisting OCD that will be of lifelong benefit.

### What Is CBT?

The BT in CBT stands for behavior therapy. Behavior therapy helps people learn to change their thoughts and feelings by first changing their behavior. Behavior therapy for OCD involves *exposure* and *response prevention* (E/RP).

• *Exposure* is based on the fact that anxiety usually goes down after long enough contact with something feared. Thus people with obsessions about germs are told to stay in contact with "germy" objects (e.g., handling money) until their anxiety is extinguished. The person's anxiety tends to decrease after repeated exposure until he no longer fears the contact.

• For exposure to be of the most help, it needs to be combined with *response or ritual prevention* (RP). In RP, the person's rituals or avoidance behaviors are blocked. For example, those with excessive worries about germs must not only stay in contact with "germy things," but must also refrain from ritualized washing.

Exposure is generally more helpful in decreasing anxiety and obsessions, while response prevention is more helpful in decreasing compulsive behaviors. Despite years of struggling with OCD symptoms, many people have surprisingly little difficulty tolerating E/RP once they get started.

• *Cognitive therapy* (CT) is the other component in CBT. CT is often added to E/RP to help reduce the catastrophic thinking and exaggerated sense of responsibility often seen in those with OCD. For example, a teenager with OCD may believe that his failure to remind his mother to wear a seat belt will cause her to die that day in a car accident. CT can help him challenge the faulty assumptions in this obsession. Armed with this proof, he will be better able to engage in E/RP, for example, by not calling her at work to make sure she arrived safely.

• Other techniques, such as thought stopping and distraction (suppressing or "switching off" OCD symptoms), satiation (prolonged listening to an obsession usually using a closed-loop audiotape), habit reversal (replacing an OCD ritual with a similar but non-OCD behavior), and contingency management (using rewards and costs as incentives for ritual prevention) may sometimes be helpful but are generally less effective than standard CBT.

People react differently to psychotherapy, just as they do to medicine. CBT is relatively free of side effects, but all patients will have some anxiety during treatment. CBT can be individual (you and your doctor), group (with other people), or family. A physician may provide both CBT and medication, or a psychologist or social worker may provide CBT, while a physician manages your medications. Regardless of their specialties, those treating you should be knowledgeable about the treatment of OCD and willing to cooperate in providing your care.

## How to Get the Most Out of Psychotherapy

• Keep your appointments.
• Be honest and open.
• Do the homework assigned to you as part of your therapy.
• Give the therapist feedback on how the treatment is working.

## Commonly Asked Questions about CBT

- *How successful is CBT?* While as many as 25% of patients refuse CBT, those who complete CBT report a 50–80% reduction in OCD symptoms after 12–20 sessions. Just as important, people with OCD who respond to CBT stay well for years to come. When someone is being treated with medication, using CBT with the medication may help prevent relapse when the medication is stopped.

- *How long does CBT take to work?* When administered on a weekly basis, CBT may take 2 months or more to show its full effects. Intensive CBT, which involves 2–3 hours of therapist-assisted E/RP daily for 3 weeks, is the fastest treatment available for OCD.

- *What is the best setting for CBT?* Most patients do well with gradual weekly CBT, in which they practice in the office with the therapist once a week and then do daily E/RP homework. Homework is necessary because the situations or objects that trigger OCD are unique to the individual's environment and often cannot be reproduced in the therapist's office. In intensive CBT, the therapist may come to the patient's home or workplace to conduct E/RP sessions. On occasion, the therapist may also do this in gradual CBT. In very rare cases, when OCD is particularly severe, CBT is best conducted in a hospital setting.

- *How can I find a behavior therapist in my area?* Depending on where you live, finding a trained cognitive-behavioral psychotherapist may be difficult, especially one trained to work with children and adolescents. To locate a therapist skilled in CBT for OCD, you may want to ask your physician or other healthcare provider, an academic psychiatry or psychology department, your local OCD support group, or the Obsessive Compulsive Foundation, the Anxiety Disorders Association of America, or the Association for the Advancement of Behavioral Therapy (addresses and phone numbers are given at the end of this handout). In some cases, you may find that a local cognitive-behavioral psychotherapist has experience with depression or other anxiety disorders, but not with OCD. However, using one of the excellent treatment manuals now available, it is relatively easy to translate CBT skills from another disorder to OCD. So if there is no one immediately available, look for a skilled psychologist or psychiatrist who is willing to learn. Remember though, if you are not getting real CBT, which involves exposure and response prevention using a list of OCD symptoms that are ranked from most difficult to easiest to resist, you are probably not getting the treatment you need. Don't be afraid to ask for a second opinion where necessary. In rare cases, traveling to a specialized center where intensive CBT is available on an outpatient or inpatient basis may be the most practical solution.

## MEDICATION

### What Medications Are Used
### to Treat Obsessive–Compulsive Disorder?

Research clearly shows that the serotonin reuptake inhibitors (SRIs) are uniquely effective treatments for OCD. These medications increase the concentration of serotonin, a chemical messenger in the brain. Five SRIs are currently available by prescription in the United States:

- Clomipramine (Anafranil, manufactured by Ciba-Geigy)
- Fluoxetine (Prozac, manufactured by Lilly)
- Fluvoxamine (Luvox, manufactured by Solvay)
- Paroxetine (Paxil, manufactured by SmithKline Beecham)
- Sertraline (Zoloft, manufactured by Pfizer)

Fluoxetine, fluvoxamine, paroxetine, and sertraline are called selective serotonin reuptake inhibitors (SSRIs) because they primarily affect only serotonin. Clomipramine is a nonselective SRI, which means that it affects many other neurotransmitters besides serotonin. This means that clomipramine has a more complicated set of side effects than the SSRIs. For this reason, the SSRIs are usually tried first since they are usually easier for people to tolerate.

### How Well Do Medications Work?

When patients are asked about how well they are doing compared to before starting treatment, they report marked to moderate improvement after 8–10 weeks on an SRI. Unfortunately, fewer than 20% of those treated with medication alone end up with no OCD symptoms. This is why medication is often combined with CBT to get more complete and lasting results. About 20% don't experience much improvement with the first SRI and need to try another SRI.

### Which Medication Should I Choose First?

Studies show that all the SRIs are about equally effective. However, to reduce the chance of side effects, most experts recommend beginning treatment with one of the SSRIs. If you or someone in your family did well or poorly with a medication in the past, this may influence the choice. If you have medical problems (e.g., an irritable stomach, problems sleeping) or are taking another medication, these factors may cause your doctor to recommend one or another medication to minimize side effects or to avoid possible drug interactions.

## What If the First Medication Doesn't Work?

First, it is important to remember that these medications don't work right away. Most patients notice some benefit after 3 to 4 weeks, while maximum benefit should occur after 10 to 12 weeks of treatment at an adequate dose of medication. When it is clear that a medication is not working well enough, most experts recommend switching to another SRI. While most patients do equally well on any of the SRIs, some will do better on one than another, so it is important to keep trying until you find the medication and dosage schedule that is right for you.

## What Are the Side Effects of These Medications?

In general, the SRIs are well tolerated by most people with OCD. The four SSRIs (fluoxetine, fluvoxamine, paroxetine, and sertraline) have similar side effects. These include nervousness, insomnia, restlessness, nausea, and diarrhea. The most common side effects of clomipramine are dry mouth, sedation, dizziness, and weight gain. While all five drugs can cause sexual problems, on average these are a bit more common with clomipramine. Clomipramine is also more likely to cause problems with blood pressure and irregular heart beats, so that children and adolescents and patients with preexisting heart disease who are treated with clomipramine must have electrocardiograms before beginning treatment and at regular intervals during treatment. Remember that all side effects depend on the dose of medication and on how long you have been taking it. If side effects are a big issue, it is important to start with a low dose and increase the dose slowly. More severe side effects are associated with larger doses and a rapid increase in the dose. Tolerance to side effects may be more likely to develop with the SSRIs than with clomipramine, so that many patients are better able to tolerate the SSRIs than clomipramine over the long term. All SRIs except fluoxetine should be tapered and stopped slowly because of the possibility of the return of symptoms and withdrawal reactions.

## Tell Your Doctor Right Away about Any Side Effects You Have

Some people have different side effects than others and one person's side effect (for example, unpleasant sleepiness) may actually help another person (someone with insomnia). The side effects you may get from medication depend on:

- The type and amount of medicine you take
- Your body chemistry
- Your age
- Other medicines you are taking
- Other medical conditions you have

If side effects are a problem for you, your doctor can try a number of things to help:

- Reducing the amount of medicine: The doctor may gradually lower the dose to try to achieve a dose low enough to reduce side effects but not low enough to cause a relapse.
- Adding another medication may be helpful for some side effects, such as trouble sleeping or sexual problems.
- Trying a different medicine to see if there are fewer or less bothersome side effects: Even when a medication is clearly helping, side effects sometimes make it intolerable. In such a case, trying another SRI is a reasonable strategy.

Remember: Changing medicine is a complicated, potentially risky decision. Don't stop your medicine or change the dose on your own. Discuss any medication problems you are having with your doctor.

## Does It Help to Add CBT or Another Medication to an SRI?

When medication has produced only a little benefit after 6 weeks, adding CBT or another medication to the SRI is also sometimes useful.

Many experts believe that CBT is the most helpful treatment to add when someone with OCD is not responding well to medication alone. When people continue to avoid the things that make them anxious or continue to do rituals, this blocks the effects of the medication. For the medication to work, therefore, the person with OCD must try to resist doing rituals. Adding CBT to medication is helpful because it teaches those with OCD to expose themselves to the triggers that make them anxious and then to resist performing rituals.

It may also be helpful to add one of the following types of medications to an SRI:

- Low dose clomipramine to an SSRI
- An anxiety-reducing medication, such as clonazepam or alprazolam, in patients with high levels of anxiety
- A high potency neuroleptic, such as haloperidol or risperidone, when tics or thought-disorder symptoms are present.

These complex medication strategies are best reserved for those who have not done well with a combination of SRI and CBT.

## What If Nothing Seems to Work?

Before deciding that a treatment has failed, your therapist needs to be sure that the treatment has been given in a large enough dose for a sufficient period of time. There is little consensus among the OCD experts on what to do next when someone with OCD fails to respond to expert CBT plus well-delivered, sequential SRI trials. Switching from an SSRI to clomipramine may improve the chances that a previously nonresponsive patient may have a good response. Most experts recommend considering a trial of clomipramine after 2 or 3 failed SSRI trials. Occasionally, a doctor may wish to combine an SSRI with clomipramine either to reduce side effects or to increase the potential benefits of medication. In the adult with extremely severe and unremitting OCD, neurosurgical treatment to interrupt specific brain circuits that are malfunctioning can be very helpful. In patients who have severe OCD and depression, electroconvulsive therapy (ECT) may be of benefit.

## Answers to Other Questions about Medications

- If you think you might be pregnant or are planning to become pregnant, most experts prefer to treat OCD with CBT alone. However, if medications are necessary (and they may be since OCD commonly gets worse during pregnancy), it is better to use them sparingly and to select an SSRI rather than clomipramine.
- The SSRIs are preferred in patients with renal failure or coexisting heart disease who require medication,.
- When another psychiatric disorder is present, your doctor will likely mix and match treatment for the other conditions with treatment for OCD. Sometimes, the same medication can be used for two disorders (e.g., an SRI for OCD and panic disorder). In other cases, such as concurrent mania and OCD, more than one medication will be necessary (e.g., a mood stabilizer and an SRI).

- Laboratory tests are necessary before and during treatment with clomipramine, but not with the SSRIs.
- The SRIs are not addictive, but it is a good idea to stop them gradually.

## Is Hospitalization an Option?

People with OCD can almost always be treated as outpatients. In very rare cases in which the OCD involves severe depression or aggressive impulses, hospitalization may be necessary for safety. When a person has very severe OCD or the OCD is complicated by a medical or neuropsychiatric illness, hospitalization can sometimes be a useful way to give intensive CBT.

## Do I Have to Choose between CBT and Medication?

No single approach works best for everyone with OCD, although most people probably do best with CBT alone or CBT plus an SRI. The treatment choice will of course depend on the patient's preference. Some people prefer to start with medication to avoid the time and trouble associated with CBT; others prefer to begin with CBT to avoid medication side effects. Many, if not most, people seem to prefer combination treatment.

The need for medication depends on the severity of the OCD and the age of the person. In milder OCD, CBT alone is often the initial choice, but medication may also be needed if CBT is not effective enough. Individuals with severe OCD or complicating conditions that may interfere with CBT (e.g., panic disorder, depression) often need to start with medication, adding CBT once the medicine has provided some relief. In younger patients, clinicians are more likely to use CBT alone. However, trained cognitive-behavioral psychotherapists are in short supply. Thus, when CBT is not available, medication may become the treatment of choice. Consequently, it is likely that many more people with OCD receive medication than CBT.

Before deciding on a treatment approach, you and your clinician will need to assess your OCD symptoms, other disorders you have, the availability of CBT, and your wishes and desires about what treatment you want. Try to find a clinician who will talk to you about these possibilities so that you can make your own best choice among the options available to you.

## What If I Belong to a Managed Care Network?

More and more people in the United States are receiving their medical care in some kind of managed care setting (HMO, preferred provider organization, etc.). If you have OCD, it is important that you talk to your case manager or administrator to find out what types of therapy are available in your network. Many managed care programs are instituting group therapy programs as a means of providing appropriate treatment at an affordable cost.

## What If I Can't Afford the Medications?

The companies who manufacture the five SRI medications listed above each have a special program to provide free medications for patients who cannot afford them. The Pharmaceutical Research and Manufacturers Association publishes a directory of programs for those who cannot afford medications, which your doctor can request by calling 202-835-3450. You or your doctor can also contact the companies directly:

- Ciba-Geigy Patient Support Program: 800-257-3273
- Lilly Cares Program: 800-545-6962
- Pfizer Prescription Assistance: 800-646-4455
- SmithKline Paxil Access to Care Program: 800-546-0420 (patient requests); 215-751-5722 (physician requests)
- Solvay Patient Assistance Program: 800-788-9277

## MAINTENANCE TREATMENT

Once OCD symptoms are eliminated or much reduced—a goal which is practical for the majority of those with OCD—then maintenance of treatment gains becomes the goal.

## Maintaining Treatment Gains

- When patients have completed a successful course of treatment for OCD, most experts recommend monthly follow-up visits for at least 6 months and continued treatment for at least 1 year before trying to stop medications or CBT.
- Relapse is very common when medication is withdrawn, particularly if the person has not had the benefit of CBT. Therefore, many experts recommend that patients continue medication if they do not have access to CBT.
- Individuals who have repeated episodes of OCD may need to receive long-term or even lifelong prophylactic medication. The experts recommend such long-term treatment after 2 to 4 severe relapses or 3 to 4 milder relapses.

Discontinuing Treatment

• When someone has done well with maintenance treatment and does not need long-term medication, most experts suggest discontinuing medication only very gradually, while giving CBT booster sessions to prevent relapse. Gradual medication withdrawal usually involves lowering the dose by 25% and then waiting 2 months before lowering it again, depending on how the person responds.

• Because OCD is a lifetime waxing and waning condition, you should always feel comfortable returning to your clinician if your OCD symptoms come back.

## SUPPORT GROUPS

Support groups are an invaluable part of treatment. These groups provide a forum for mutual acceptance, understanding, and self-discovery. Participants develop a sense of camaraderie with other attendees because they have all lived with OCD. People new to OCD can talk to others who have learned successful strategies for coping with the illness.

The Obsessive–Compulsive Foundation (OCF) provides a forum for people with OCD and professionals interested in OCD. It distributes information and helps sponsor research on the nature and treatment of OCD and some related conditions. The OCF has self-help groups in many parts of the country and provides referrals to therapists, clinics, and self-help groups. OCF conducts an annual meeting at which the latest findings about OCD are presented and has recently begun training institutes to try to make CBT more widely available. Membership includes a newsletter and discounts for the annual meeting and OCF materials.

Obsessive–Compulsive Foundation
P.O. Box 70
Milford, CT 06460-0070
203-878-5669
203-874-3843 (recorded information)

You may wish to visit the OC Foundation's website: http://pages.prodigy.com/alwillen/ocf.html, where you'll find a list of other OCD resources on the WWW as well as lots of useful information about OCD.

The Obsessive–Compulsive Information Center is staffed by medical librarians. It provides access to the published literature on OCD and publishes very useful guides concerning OCD and some related disorders, such as trichotillomania.

OC Information Center
2711 Allen Boulevard
Middleton, WI 53562
608-836-8070

The Anxiety Disorders Association of America provides a central clearinghouse for people with, and professionals interested in, the diagnosis and treatment of all anxiety disorders, including OCD.

Anxiety Disorders Association of America
6000 Executive Boulevard, Suite 513
Rockville, MD 20852
301-231-9350

The Tourette Syndrome Association (TSA) provides a central clearinghouse for people with, and professionals interested in, the diagnosis and treatment of tic disorders. Because tic disorders often overlap with OCD, the TSA has a wealth of information about the overlap between these two conditions.

Tourette Syndrome Association
42-40 Bell Boulevard
New York, NY 11361-2874
718-224-2999

Association for Advancement of Behavior Therapy

305 Seventh Avenue, 16th Floor
New York, NY 10001-6008
212-647-1890

## FOR MORE INFORMATION

Most of the following materials are available from the OC Foundation.

Baer, L. (1991). *Getting control*. Little, Brown.

Callner, J. (1994). *The touching tree: A video about a young child with OCD*. Available through the OC Foundation, P.O. Box 70, Milford, CT 06460-0070.

Ciarrocchi, J. (1995). *The doubting disease*. Paulist Press.

Foa, E., & Wilson, R. (1991). *Stop obsessing!* Bantam.

Greist, J. (1994). *Obsessive compulsive disorder: A guide* (2nd ed.). Obsessive Compulsive Information Center.

Johnston, H. F. (1993). *Obsessive–compulsive disorder in children and adolescents.* Obsessive–Compulsive Information Center.

March, J., Frances, A., Carpenter, D., & Kahn, D. (1997) The expert consensus guideline series: Treatment of obsessive–compulsive disorder. *Journal of Clinical Psychiatry, 58*(Suppl. 4).

Neziroglu, F., & Yaryura-Tobias, J. A. (1995). *Over and over again: Understanding obsessive compulsive disorder* (2nd ed.). Lexington Books.

Rapoport, J. (1991). *The boy who couldn't stop washing.* Penguin Books.

Schwartz, J. (1996). *Brain lock.* Harper Collins.

Steketee, G., & White, K. (1990). *When once is not enough: Help for obsessive–compulsives.* Harbinger Publications.

VanNoppen, B., Pato, M., & Rasmussen, S. (1997). *Learning to live with obsessive compulsive disorder* (4th ed.). Milford.

## TO REQUEST MORE COPIES OF THIS HANDOUT

Please contact the OC Foundation, visit the EKS website (www.psychguides.com), or write:

Expert Knowledge Systems, L.L.C.
P.O. Box 917
Independence, VA 24348

# References

Adams, G. B., Waas, G. A., March, J. S., & Smith, M. C. (1994). Obsessive compulsive disorder in children and adolescents: The role of the school psychologist in identification, assessment, and treatment. *School Psychology Quarterly, 9*(4), 274–294.

Albano, A. M., Knox, L. S., & Barlow, D. H. (1995). *Obsessive–compulsive disorder.* Northvale, NJ: Jason Aronson.

Allen, A. J., Leonard, H. L., & Swedo, S. E. (1995). Case study: A new infection-triggered, autoimmune subtype of pediatric OCD and Tourette's syndrome. *Journal of the American Academy of Child and Adolescent Psychiatry, 34*(3), 307–311.

American Psychiatric Association. (1994). *Diagnostic and statistical manual of mental disorders* (4th ed.). Washington, DC: Author.

Apter, A., Ratzioni, G., & King, R. (1994). Fluxoxamine open-lablel treatment of adolescent inpatients with obsessive–compulsive disorder or depression. *Journal of the American Academy of Child and Adolescent Psychiatry, 33,* 342–348.

Baer, L. (1991). *Getting control.* Boston: Little, Brown.

Baer, L. (1992). Behavior therapy for obsessive–compulsive disorder and trichotillomania: Implications for Tourette syndrome. *Advances in Neurology, 58*(333), 333–340.

Baer, L., Jenike, M. A., Black, D. W., Treece, C., Rosenfeld, R., & Greist, J. (1992). Effect of axis II diagnoses on treatment outcome with clomipramine in 55 patients with obsessive–compulsive disorder. *Archives of General Psychiatry, 49*(11), 862–866.

Barkley, R. A. (1995) *Taking charge of ADHD.* New York: Guilford Press.

Barlow, D. H. (1992). Cognitive-behavioral approaches to panic disorder and social phobia. *Bulletin of the Menninger Clinic, 56*(2, Suppl. A), A14–A28.

Barlow, D., & Craske, M. (1989). *Mastery of your anxiety and panic.* Albany, NY: Graywind.

Barr, L. C., Goodman, W. K., Price, L. H., McDougle, C. J., & Charney, D. S. (1992). The serotonin hypothesis of obsessive compulsive disorder: Implications of pharmacologic challenge studies. *Journal of Clinical Psychiatry, 53,* 17–28.

Baxter, L. J., Schwartz, J. M., Bergman, K. S., Szuba, M. P., Guze, B. H., Mazziotta, J. C., Alazraki, A., Selin, C. E., Ferng, H. K., Munford, P., et al. (1992). Caudate glucose metabolic rate changes with both drug and behavior therapy for obsessive–compulsive disorder. *Archives of General Psychiatry, 49*(9), 681–689.

Berg, C., Rapoport, J., & Wolff, R. (1989). Behavioral treatment for obsessive–compulsive disorder in childhood. In J. Rapoport (Ed.), *Obsessive–compulsive disorder in children and adolescents* (pp. 169–185). Washington, DC: American Psychiatric Press.

Berg, C. Z., Whitaker, A., Davies, M., Flament, M. F., & Rapoport, J. L. (1988). The survey form of the Leyton Obsessional Inventory—Child Version: Norms from an epidemiological study. *Journal of the American Academy of Child and Adolescent Psychiatry, 27*(6), 759–763.

Clark, D. (1982). Primary obsessional slowness: A nursing treatment programme with a 13 year old male adolescent. *Behaviour Research Therapy, 20*(3), 289–292.

Clarkin, J. F., & Kendall, P. C. (1992). Comorbidity and treatment planning: Summary and future directions. *Journal of Consulting and Clinical Psychology, 60*(6), 904–908.

Cohen, D. J., & Leckman, J. F. (1994). Developmental psychopathology and neurobiology of Tourette's syndrome [Review]. *Journal of the American Academy of Child and Adolescent Psychiatry, 33*(1), 2–15.

Conners, C. (1995). *Conners' Rating Scales.* Toronto: MultiHealth Systems.

Conners, C. K., & March, J. S. (1996). *Conners–March Developmental Questionnaire.* Toronto: MultiHealth Systems.

Cook, E., Charak, D., Trapani, C., & Zelko, F. (1994). Sertraline treatment of obsessive–compulsive disorder in children and adolescents: Preliminary findings. *Scientific Proceeding of the AACAP Annual Meeting,* New York, 57–58.

Cox, C., Fedio, P., & Rapoport, J. (1989). Neuropsychological testing of obsessive–compulsive adolescents. In J. Rapoport (Ed.), *Obsessive–compulsive disorder in children and adolescents* (pp. 73–86). Washington, DC: American Psychiatric Press.

Dar, R., & Greist, J. H. (1992). Behavior therapy for obsessive compulsive disorder. *Psychiatric Clinics of North America, 15*(4), 885–894.

Denckla, M. (1989). Neurological examination. In J. Rapoport (Ed.), *Obsessive–compulsive disorder in children and adolescents* (pp. 107–118). Washington, DC: American Psychiatric Press.

DeVeaugh-Geiss, J., Katz, R., Landau, P., & Moroz, G. (1991). *Clomipramine hydrochloride (Anafranil) in the treatment of obsessive–compulsive disorder: Results from three multicentre trials.* Bern, Switzerland: Hogrefe & Huber.

DeVeaugh-Geiss, J., Moroz, G., Biederman, J., Cantwell, D., Fontaine, R., Greist, J. H., Reichler, R., Katz, R., & Landau, P. (1992). Clomipramine hydrochloride in childhood and adolescent obsessive–compulsive disorder—A multicenter trial. *Journal of the American Academy of Child and Adolescent Psychiatry*, *31*(1), 45–49.

Elliott, G., & Popper, C. (1991). Tricyclic antidepressants: The QT interval and other cardiovascular parameters. *Journal of Child and Adolescent Psychopharmacology*, *1*, 187–191.

Emmelkamp, P., Bouman, T., & Scholing, A. (1989). *Anxiety disorders: A practitioner's guide*. West Sussex, England: Wiley.

Esman, A. (1989). Psychoanalysis in general psychiatry: Obsessive–compulsive disorder as a paradigm. *Journal of the American Psychoanalytical Association*, *37*, 319–336.

Flament, M. (1990). Epidemiology of obsessive–compulsive disorder in children and adolescents [French]. *Encephale*, *16*, 311–316.

Flament, M. F., Rapoport, J. L., Berg, C. J., Sceery, W., Kilts, C., Mellstrom, B., & Linnoila, M. (1985). Clomipramine treatment of childhood obsessive–compulsive disorder: A double-blind controlled study. *Archives of General Psychiatry*, *42*(10), 977–983.

Flament, M. F., Whitaker, A., Rapoport, J. L., Davies, M., Berg, C. Z., Kalikow, K., Sceery, W., & Shaffer, D. (1988). Obsessive compulsive disorder in adolescence: An epidemiological study. *Journal of the American Academy of Child and Adolescent Psychiatry*, *27*(6), 764–771.

Foa, E., & Emmelkamp, P. (1983). *Failures in behavior therapy*. New York: Wiley.

Foa, E., & Kozak, M. (1985). Emotional processing of fear: Exposure to corrective information. *Psychological Bulletin*, *90*, 20–35.

Foa, E. B., Rothbaum, B. O., & Kozak, M. J. (1989). Behavioral treatments for anxiety and depression. In P. Kendall & D. Watson (Eds.), *Personality, psychopathology, and psychotherapy* (pp. 413–454). San Diego, CA: Academic Press.

Foa, E., & Wilson, R. (1991). *Stop obsessing!* New York: Bantam.

Gesell, A., Ames, L., & Ilg, F. (1974). *Infant and child in the culture today*. New York: Harper and Row.

Goleman, D. (1976). Meditation and consciousness: An Asian approach to mental health. *American Journal of Psychotherapy*, *30*(1), 41–54.

Goodman, W. K., & Price, L. H. (1992). Assessment of severity and change in obsessive compulsive disorder. *Psychiatric Clinics of North America*, *15*(4), 861–869.

Goodman, W. K., Price, L. H., Rasmussen, S. A., Delgado, P. L., Heninger, G. R., & Charney, D. S. (1989). Efficacy of fluvoxamine in obsessive–compulsive disorder. A double-blind comparison with placebo. *Archives of General Psychiatry*, *46*(1), 36–44.

Goodman, W. K., Price, L. H., Rasmussen, S. A., Mazure, C., Delgado, P.,

Heninger, G. R., & Charney, D. S. (1989). The Yale–Brown Obsessive Compulsive Scale: II. Validity. *Archives of General Psychiatry, 46(11)*, 1012–1016.

Goodman, W. K., Price, L. H., Rasmussen, S. A., Mazure, C., Fleischmann, R. L., Hill, C. L., Heninger, G. R., & Charney, D. S. (1989). The Yale–Brown Obsessive Compulsive Scale: I. Development, use, and reliability. *Archives of General Psychiatry, 46*(11), 1006–1011.

Goodman, W., Rasmussen, S., Foa, E., and Price, L. (1994). Obsessive–Compulsive Disorder. In R. Prien & D. Robinson (Eds.), *Clinical evaluation of psychotropic drugs: Principles and guidelines* (pp. 431–466). New York: Raven Press.

Greist, J. H., Jefferson, J. W., Rosenfeld, R., Gutzmann, L. D., March, J. S., & Barklage, N. E. (1990). Clomipramine and obsessive compulsive disorder: A placebo-controlled double-blind study of 32 patients. *Journal of Clinical Psychiatry, 51*(7), 292–297.

Guy, W. (1976) *ECDEU assessment manual for psychopharmacology* (2nd ed., DHEW Pub. No. ABM 76-388). Washington, DC: U. S. Government Printing Office.

Hamburger, S. D., Swedo, S., Whitaker, A., Davies, M., & Rapoport, J. L. (1989). Growth rate in adolescents with obsessive–compulsive disorder. *American Journal of Psychiatry, 146*(5), 652–655.

Hand, I. (1988). Obsessive–compulsive patients and their families. In I. R. H. Falloon (Ed.), *Handbook of behavioral family therapy* (pp. 231–256). New York: Guilford Press.

Hibbs, E. D., Hamburger, S. D., Kruesi, M. J., & Lenane, M. (1993). Factors affecting expressed emotion in parents of ill and normal children. *American Journal of Orthopsychiatry, 63*(1), 103–112.

Hibbs, E. D., Hamburger, S. D., Lenane, M., Rapoport, J. L., Kruesi, M. J., Keysor, C. S., & Goldstein, M. J. (1991). Determinants of expressed emotion in families of disturbed and normal children. *Journal of Child Psychology and Psychiatry and Allied Disciplines, 32*(5), 757–770.

Hollander, E., Schiffman, E., Cohen, B., Rivera, S. M., Rosen, W., Gorman, J. M., Fyer, A. J., Papp, L., & Liebowitz, M. R. (1990). Signs of central nervous system dysfunction in obsessive–compulsive disorder. *Archives of General Psychiatry, 47*(1), 27–32.

Hymas, N., Lees, A., Bolton, D., Epps, K., & Head, D. (1991). The neurology of obsessional slowness. *Brain, 114(5)*, 2203–2233.

Janet, P. (1903). *Les obsessions et la psychiatrie* (Vol. 1). Paris: Felix Alan.

Jenike, M. A. (1989). Obsessive–compulsive and related disorders: A hidden epidemic [Editorial; comment]. *New England Journal of Medicine, 321*(8), 539–541.

Jenike, M. A. (1992). Pharmacologic treatment of obsessive compulsive disorders. *Psychiatric Clinics of North America, 15(4)*, 895–919.

Jenike, M., & Rauch, S. (1994). Managing the patient with treatment resistant obsessive compulsive disorder: Current strategies. *Journal of Clinical Psychiatry, 55*(Suppl. 3), 11–17.

Johnston, H., & March, J. (1993). Obsessive–compulsive disorder in children and adolescents. In W. Reynolds (Ed.), *Internalizing disorders in children and adolescents* (pp. 107–148). New York: Wiley.

Kahn, D. A., Carpenter, D., Docherty, J. P., & Frances, A. (1996). The Expert Consensus Guideline Series: Treatment of bipolar disorder. *Journal of Clinical Psychiatry, 57*(Suppl. 12A).

Katz, R. J., DeVeaugh, G. J., & Landau, P. (1990). Clomipramine in obsessive–compulsive disorder. *Biological Psychiatry, 28*(5), 401–414.

Kettl, P., & Marks, I. (1986). Neurological factors in obsessive–compulsive disorder. *British Journal of Psychiatry, 149,* 315–319.

Kiessling, L. S., Marcotte, A. C., & Culpepper, L. (1994). Antineuronal antibodies: Tics and obsessive–compulsive symptoms. *Journal of Developmental Behavioral Pediatrics, 15*(6), 421–425.

Lenane, M. (1989). Families in obsessive–compulsive disorder. In J. Rapoport (Ed.), *Obsessive–compulsive disorder in children and adolescents* (pp. 237–249). Washington, DC: American Psychiatric Press.

Leonard, H. L., Goldberger, E. L., Rapoport, J. L., Cheslow, D. L., & Swedo, S. E. (1990). Childhood rituals: Normal development or obsessive–compulsive symptoms? *Journal of the American Academy of Child and Adolescent Psychiatry, 29*(1), 17–23.

Leonard, H., Lenane, M., & Swedo, S. (1993). Obsessive–compulsive disorder. In H. L. Leonard (Ed.), *Child psychiatric clinics of North America: Anxiety disorders* (Vol. 2, pp. 655–666). New York: Saunders.

Leonard, H. L., Lenane, M. C., Swedo, S. E., Rettew, D. C., Gershon, E. S., & Rapoport, J. L. (1992). Tics and Tourette's disorder: a 2- to 7-year follow-up of 54 obsessive–compulsive children. *American Journal of Psychiatry, 149*(9), 1244–1251.

Leonard, H. L., Lenane, M. C., Swedo, S. E., Rettew, D. C., & Rapoport, J. L. (1991). A double-blind comparison of clomipramine and desipramine treatment of severe onychophagia (nail biting). *Archives of General Psychiatry, 48*(9), 821–827.

Leonard, H. L., Meyer M. C., et al. (1995). Electrocardiographic changes during desipramine and clomipramine treatment in children and adolescents. *Journal of the American Academy of Child and Adolescent Psychiatry 34*(11), 1460–1468.

Leonard, H. L., & Rapoport, J. L. (1989). Pharmacotherapy of childhood obsessive–compulsive disorder. *Psychiatric Clinics of North America, 12*(4), 963–970.

Leonard, H. L., Swedo, S. E., Lenane, M. C., Rettew, D. C., Cheslow, D. L., Hamburger, S. D., & Rapoport, J. L. (1991). A double-blind desipramine substitution during long-term clomipramine treatment in children and adolescents with obsessive–compulsive disorder. *Archives of General Psychiatry, 48*(10), 922–927.

Leonard, H. L., Swedo, S. E., Lenane, M. C., Rettew, D. C., Hamburger, S. D., Bartko, J. J., & Rapoport, J. L. (1993). A 2- to 7-year follow-up study of 54 obsessive–compulsive children and adolescents. *Archives of General Psychiatry, 50*(6), 429–439.

Leonard, H. L., Swedo, S. E., Rapoport, J. L., Koby, E. V., Lenane, M. C., Cheslow, D. L., & Hamburger, S. D. (1989). Treatment of obsessive–compulsive disorder with clomipramine and desipramine in children and adolescents. A double-blind crossover comparison. *Archives of General Psychiatry, 46*(12), 1088–1092.

Leonard, H., Topol, D., Swedo, S., Bukstein, O., Hindmarsh, D., & Allen, A. (1995). Clonazepam as an augmenting agent in the treatment of childhood-onset obsessive–compulsive disorder. *Journal of the American Academy of Child and Adolescent Psychiatry, 33*(6), 792–794.

Lewinsohn, P. M., Clarke, G. N., & Rohde, P. (1994). *Psychological approaches to the treatment of depression in adolescents.* New York: Plenum.

March, J. S. (1995). Cognitive-behavioral psychotherapy for children and adolescents with OCD: A review and recommendations for treatment. *Journal of the American Academy of Child and Adolescent Psychiatry, 34*(1), 7–18.

March, J., & Albano, A. (1996). Assessment of anxiety in children and adolescents. In L. Dickstein, M. Riba, & M. Oldham (Eds.), *Review of psychiatry XV* (pp. 405–427). Washington, DC: American Psychiatric Press.

March, J., Biederman, J., Wolkow, R., Safferman, A., and Group, S. S. (1997). *Sertraline in children and adolescents with obsessive compulsive disorder: A multicenter double-blind placebo-controlled study.* Paper presented at the annual meeting of the American Psychiatric Association, San Diego, CA.

March, J., Frances, A., Carpenter, D., & Kahn, D. (1997) The Expert Consensus Guideline Series: Treatment of obsessive–compulsive disorder. *Journal of Clinical Psychiatry, 58*(Suppl. 4).

March, J., Johnston, H., & Greist, J. (1990). The future of research in obsessive–compulsive disorder. In M. Jenike, L. Baer, & W. Minichello (Eds.), *Obsessive–compulsive disorder* (2nd ed., pp. 349–363). Littleton, MA: PSG.

March, J., Johnston, H., Jefferson, J., Greist, J., Kobak, K., & Mazza, J. (1990). Do subtle neurological impairments predict treatment resistance in children and adolescents with obsessive–compulsive disorder. *Journal of Child and Adolescent Psychopharmacology, 1,* 133–140.

March, J. S., Leonard, H. L., & Swedo, S. E. (1995). Pharmacotherapy of obsessive–compulsive disorder. In M. Riddle (Ed.), *Child and Adolescent Psychiatric Clinics of North America, 4*(1), 217–236.

March, J., Leonard, H., & Swedo, S. (in press). Neuropsychiatry of pediatric obsessive compulsive disorder. In E. Coffey & R. Brumback (Eds.), *Textbook of pediatric neuropsychiatry.* Washington, DC: American Psychiatric Press.

March, J., & Mulle, K. (1995). Manualized cognitive-behavioral psychotherapy for obsessive–compulsive disorder in childhood: A preliminary single case study. *Journal of Anxiety Disorders, 9*(2), 175–184.

March, J., & Mulle, K. (1996). Banishing obsessive–compulsive disorder. In E. Hibbs & P. Jensen (Eds.), *Psychosocial treatments for child and adolescent disorders* (pp. 82–103). Washington, DC: American Psychological Press.

March, J., Mulle, K., & Herbel, B. (1994). Behavioral psychotherapy for children and adolescents with obsessive–compulsive disorder: An open trial of a new protocol driven treatment package. *Journal of the American Academy of Child and Adolescent Psychiatry, 33*(3), 333–341.

March, J., Mulle, K., Stallings, P., Erhardt, D., & Conners, C. (1995). Organizing an anxiety disorders clinic. In J. March (Ed.), *Anxiety disorders in children and adolescents* (pp. 420–435). New York: Guilford Press.

March, J., Wells, K., & Conners, C. (1995). Attention-deficit/hyperactivity disorder: Part I. Assessment and diagnosis. *Journal of Practical Psychiatry and Behavioral Health, 1*(4), 219–228.

March, J., Wells, K., & Conners, C. (1996). Attention-deficit/hyperactivity disorder: Part II. Treatment. *Journal of Practical Psychiatry and Behavioral Health, 2*(1), 23–32.

Marks, I. (1987). *Fears, phobias, and rituals.* New York: Oxford University Press.

Marks, I., Hodgson, R., & Rachman, S. (1975). Treatment of chronic obsessive–compulsive neurosis by in vivo exposure. *British Journal of Psychiatry, 127,* 349–364.

Marks, I. M., Lelliott, P., Basoglu, M., Noshirvani, H., Monteiro, W., Cohen, D., & Kasvikis, Y. (1988). Clomipramine, self-exposure and therapist-aided exposure for obsessive–compulsive rituals. *British Journal of Psychiatry, 152,* 522–534.

McDougle, C., Goodman, W., Leckman, J., Lee, N., Heninger, G., & Price, L. (1994). Haloperidol addition in fluvoxamine-refractory obsessive–compulsive disorder. *Archives of General Psychiatry, 51,* 302–308.

McEvoy, J. P., Weiden, P. J., Smith, T. E., Carpenter, D., Kahn, D. A., & Frances, A. (1996). The Expert Consensus Guideline Series: Treatment of schizophrenia. *Journal of Clinical Psychiatry, 57*(Suppl. 12B), 1–58.

Miller, J. J., Fletcher, K., & Kabat-Zinn, J. (1995). Three-year follow-up and clinical implications of a mindfulness meditation-based stress reduction intervention in the treatment of anxiety disorders. *General Hospital Psychiatry, 17*(3), 192–200.

Neziroglu, F., & Neuman, J. (1990). Three treatment approaches for obsessions. *Journal of Cognitive Psychotherapy, 4*(4), 377–392.

Pauls, D. L., Alsobrook, J. P., Goodman, W., Rasmussen, S., & Leckman J. (1995). A family study of obsessive–compulsive disorder. *American Journal of Psychiatry, 152*(1), 76–84.

Pauls, D., Towbin, K., Leckman, J., Zahner, G., & Cohen, D. (1986). Gilles de la Tourette syndrome and obsessive compulsive disorder: Evidence supporting a genetic relationship. *Archives of General Psychiatry, 43,* 1180–1182.

Peterson, A. L., Campise, R. L., & Azrin, N. H. (1994). Behavioral and pharmacological treatments for tic and habit disorders: A review. *Journal of Developmental Behavioral Pediatrics, 15(6),* 430–441.

Piacentini, J., Gitow, A., Jaffer, M., & Graae, F. (1994). Outpatient behavioral treatment of child and adolescent obsessive compulsive disorder. *Journal of Anxiety Disorders, 8(3),* 277–289.

Piacentini, J., Jaffer, M., Gitow, A., Graae, F., Davies, S. O., Del, B. D., & Liebowitz, M. (1992). Psychopharmacologic treatment of child and adolescent obsessive compulsive disorder. *Psychiatric Clinics of North America, 15(1),* 87–107.

Pigott T, L'Heureux F., Rubenstein, C. (1992). *A controlled trial of clonazepam augmentation in OCD patients treated with clomipramine or fluoxetine.* Paper presented at the 145th annual meeting of the American Psychiatric Association, Washington, DC.

Rapoport, J. L. (1991). Recent advances in obsessive–compulsive disorder. *Neuropsychopharmacology, 5(1),* 1–10.

Rapoport, J. L., Leonard, H. L., Swedo, S. E., & Lenane, M. C. (1993). Obsessive compulsive disorder in children and adolescents: Issues in management. *Journal of Clinical Psychiatry, 54*(Suppl.), 27–30.

Rapoport, J. L., Swedo, S. E., & Leonard, H. L. (1992). Childhood obsessive compulsive disorder. *Journal of Clinical Psychiatry, 56,* 11–16.

Rasmussen, S. A., & Eisen, J. L. (1990). Epidemiology of obsessive compulsive disorder. *Journal of Clinical Psychiatry, 53*(Suppl.), 10–14.

Rasmussen, S. A., & Eisen, J. L. (1992). The epidemiology and differential diagnosis of obsessive compulsive disorder. *Journal of Clinical Psychiatry, 55,* 4–10.

Ratnasuriya, R. H., Marks, I. M., Forshaw, D. M., & Hymas, N. F. (1991). Obsessive slowness revisited. *British Journal of Psychiatry, 159,* 273–274.

Rauch, S. L., Jenike, M. A., Alpert, N. M., Baer, L., Breiter, H. C., Savage, C. R., & Fischman, A. J. (1994). Regional cerebral blood flow measured during symptom provocation in obsessive–compulsive disorder using oxygen 15-labeled carbon dioxide and positron emission tomography. *Archives of General Psychiatry, 51(1),* 62–70.

Rettew, D. C., Swedo, S. E., Leonard, H. L., Lenane, M. C., & Rapoport, J. L. (1992). Obsessions and compulsions across time in 79 children and adolescents with obsessive–compulsive disorder. *Journal of the American Academy of Child and Adolescent Psychiatry, 31(6),* 1050–1056.

Riddle, M., Claghorn, J., Gaffney, G., Greist, J., Holland, D., Landbloom, R., McConville, B., Pigott, T., Pravetz, M., Walkup, J., Yaryura-Tobias, J., & Houser, V. (1996). *A controlled trial of fluvoxamine for OCD in children and adolescents.* Paper presented at the NCDEU, Boca Raton, Florida

Riddle, M. A., Scahill, L., King, R. A., Hardin, M. T., Anderson, G. M., Ort,

S. I., Smith, J. C., Leckman, J. F., & Cohen, D. J. (1992). Double-blind, crossover trial of fluoxetine and placebo in children and adolescents with obsessive–compulsive disorder. *Journal of the American Academy of Child and Adolescent Psychiatry, 31*(6), 1062–1069.

Riddle, M. A., Scahill, L., King, R., Hardin, M. T., Towbin, K. E., Ort, S. I., Leckman, J. F., & Cohen, D. J. (1990). Obsessive compulsive disorder in children and adolescents: Phenomenology and family history. *Journal of the American Academy of Child and Adolescent Psychiatry, 29*(5), 766–772.

Rutter, M., Tizard, J., & Whitmore, K. (1970). *Education, health, and behavior.* London: Longmans.

Salkovskis, P. M., Westbrook, D., Davis, J., Jeavons, A., & Gledhill, A. (1997). Effects of neutralizing on intrusive thoughts: An experiment investigating the etiology of obsessive-compulsive disorder. *Behaviour Research Therapy, 35*(3), 211-219.

Scahill, L., Riddle, M., McSwiggin-Hardin, M., Ort, S., King, R., Goodman, W., Cicchetti, D., & Leckman, J. (1997). Children's Yale–Brown Obsessive Compulsive Scale: Reliability and validity. *Journal of the American Academy of Child and Adolescent Psychiatry, 36*(6), 844–852.

Schroeder, J. S., Mullin, A. V., Elliott, G. R., & Steiner, H. (1989). Cardiovascular effects of desipramine in children. *Journal of the American Academy of Child and Adolescent Psychiatry, 28*(3), 376–379.

Schwartz, J. (1996). *Brain lock.* New York: HarperCollins.

Schwartz, J. M., Stoessel, P. W., Baxter, L. R., Jr., Martin, K. M., & Phelps, M. E. (1996). Systematic changes in cerebral glucose metabolic rate after successful behavior modification treatment of obsessive–compulsive disorder. *Archives of General Psychiatry, 53*(2), 109–113.

Silverman, W. K., & Eisen, A. R. (1992). Age differences in the reliability of parent and child reports of child anxious symptomatology using a structured interview. *Journal of the American Academy of Child and Adolescent Psychiatry, 31*(1), 117–124.

Staebler, C. R., Pollard, C. A., & Merkel, W. T. (1993). Sexual history and quality of current relationships in patients with obsessive compulsive disorder: A comparison with two other psychiatric samples. *Journal of Sex and Marital Therapy, 19*(2), 147–153.

Steketee, G. (1994). Behavioral assessment and treatment planning with obsessive compulsive disorder: A review emphasizing clinical application. *Behavior Therapy, 25*(4), 613–633.

Swedo, S. (1989). Rituals and releasers: An ethological model of obsessive–compulsive disorder. In J. Rapoport (Ed.), *Obsessive–compulsive disorder in children and adolescents* (pp. 269–288). Washington, DC: American Psychiatric Press.

Swedo, S. (1993). Trichotillomania. *Psychiatric Annals, 23*(7), 402–407.

Swedo, S., Leonard, H., & Kiessling, L. (1994). Speculations on anti-neuronal antibody-mediated neuropsychiatric disorders of childhood. *Pediatrics, 93*(2), 323–326.

Swedo, S., Leonard, H., & Rapoport, J. (1990). Childhood-onset obsessive–

compulsive disorder. In M. Jenike, L. Baer, & Minichello (Eds.), *Obsessive–compulsive disorder*. Littleton, MA: PSG.

Swedo, S. E., Leonard, H. L., Schapiro, M. B., Casey, B. J., Mannheim, G. B., Lenane, M. C., & Rettew, D. C. (1993). Sydenham's chorea: Physical and psychological symptoms of St Vitus dance. *Pediatrics, 91*(4), 706–713.

Swedo, S., & Rapoport, J. (1990). Neurochemical and neuroendocrine considerations of obsessive–compulsive disorder in childhood. In W. Deutsch, A. Weizman, & R. Weizman (Eds.), *Application of basic neuroscience to child psychiatry* (pp. 275–284). New York: Plenum.

Swedo, S. E., Rapoport, J. L., Cheslow, D. L., Leonard, H. L., Ayoub, E. M., Hosier, D. M., & Wald, E. R. (1989). High prevalence of obsessive–compulsive symptoms in patients with Sydenham's chorea. *American Journal of Psychiatry, 146*(2), 246–249.

Swedo, S. E., Rapoport, J. L., Leonard, H., Lenane, M., & Cheslow, D. (1989). Obsessive–compulsive disorder in children and adolescents: Clinical phenomenology of 70 consecutive cases. *Archives of General Psychiatry, 46*(4), 335–341.

Swedo, S. E., Schapiro, M. B., Grady, C. L., Cheslow, D. L., Leonard, H. L., Kumar, A., Friedland, R., Rapoport, S. I., & Rapoport, J. L. (1989). Cerebral glucose metabolism in childhood-onset obsessive–compulsive disorder. *Archives of General Psychiatry, 46*(6), 518–523.

Tallis, F., & de Silva. P. (1992). Worry and obsessional symptoms: A correlational analysis. *Behaviour Research and Therapy, 30*(2), 103–105.

Thyer, B. A. (1991). Diagnosis and treatment of child and adolescent anxiety disorders. *Behavior Modification, 15*(3), 310–325.

Van Noppen, B., Steketee, G., McCorkle, B. H., and Pato, M. (1997). Group and multifamily behavioral treatment for obsessive compulsive disorder: A pilot study. *Journal of Anxiety Disorders, 11*(4), 431–446.

Vitulano, L. A., King, R. A., Scahill, L., & Cohen, D. J. (1992). Behavioral treatment of children and adolescents with trichotillomania. *Journal of the American Academy of Child and Adolescent Psychiatry, 31*(1), 139–146.

Warren, R., Zgourides, G., Monto, M. (1993). Self-report versions of the Yale–Brown Obsessive–Compulsive Scale: An assessment of a sample of normals. *Psychological Reports 73(2)*, 574.

Wells, K. (1995). Family therapy. In J. S. March (Ed.), *Anxiety disorders in children and adolescents* (pp. 401–419). New York: Guilford Press.

White, M. (1986). Negative explanation, restraint, and double description: A template for family therapy. *Family Process, 25*(2), 169–184.

White, M., & Epston, D. (1990). *Narrative means to therapeutic ends*. New York: Norton.

Wolff, R., & Rapoport, J. (1988). Behavioral treatment of childhood obsessive–compulsive disorder. *Behavior Modification, 12*(2), 252–266.

Wolff, R. P., & Wolff, L. S. (1991). Assessment and treatment of obsessive–compulsive disorder in children. *Behavior Modification, 15*(3), 372–393.

# Index